Developments in Genetic Hearing Impairment

Edited by
Dafydd Stephens FRCP, Andrew Read PhD and
Alessandro Martini MD

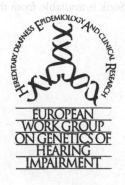

EUROPEAN
WORK GROUP
ON GENETICS OF
HEARING
IMPAIRMENT

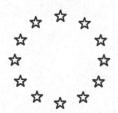

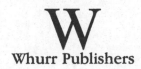

Whurr Publishers

© 1998 Whurr Publishers Ltd
First published 1998
by Whurr Publishers Ltd
19b Compton Terrace
London N1 2UN
England

British Library Cataloguing in Publication Data
A catalogue record for this book is available from the British Library.

ISBN 1 86156 058 3

Contents

Preface

This book comprises the main papers presented at the first conference on Genetic Hearing Impairment, to be held as part of the Concerted Action programme 'HEAR' under the auspices of the European Commission BIOMED 2 programme (PL 950353). The meeting was held in Milan between 11–13 October 1996.

The aims of the BIOMED 2 programme are to facilitate communication and cooperation between different groups of professionals working within the fields of genetics and of audiology and related disciplines within the EU and further afield. The programme comprises six working groups on the following topics: Definitions and audiometric investigations; Epidemiology; Vestibular function; Craniofacial disorders; Surgical management; and Clinical genetics. At the meeting in Milan, working meetings of all six study groups were held followed by public presentations by the group coordinators. A section of one of these is reported here in terms of the preliminary estimates of prevalence of genetic hearing impairment in the EU from the Epidemiology study group.

The other papers comprise a number of keynote papers given by invited speakers, with related presentations from members of the various study groups. The papers have been grouped in sections, covering general matters relevant to the field, including gene therapy and radiology, followed by a report of the development of an Internet database for use by the members of the programme and a wider audience, and decision support system for genetic hearing impairment.

The next sections are directly linked to the study groups covering the epidemiology of genetic hearing impairment, attempts to define more concise audiometric measures to use in the field, with an approach to developing a more relevant test of balance function.

These are then followed by key sections covering recessive, dominant and X-linked non-syndromal hearing impairment, starting with a keynote report of the current situation of mapping on genes resulting in non-syndromal recessive genetic hearing impairment.

A section grouping a number of papers on mitochondrial disorders reflects the growing interest in this field. This is followed by the last section covering a variety of syndromal conditions and mutations which can give rise to them.

Dafydd Stephens Andrew Read Alessandro Martini

Contributors

RJC Admiraal
University Hospital of Nijmegen, The Netherlands
LI Al-Gazali
United Arab Emirates University, Al Ain, UAE
F Amati
Tor Vergata University, Rome, Italy
AM Amodeo
University of Palermo, Italy
AR Antonelli
University of Brescia, Italy
F Apaydin
Ege University Hospital, Izmir, Turkey
B Arellano
Puerta de Hierro Hospital, Madrid, Spain
E Arslan
University of Padua, Italy
J Ashley
University of Texas Southwestern Medical Center, Dallas, Texas USA
C Barnwell
New Jersey Medical School, Newark, New Jersey USA
I. Bartolomei
Vicenza Hospital, Italy
J Bellon
Consejeria de Sanidad del Gobierno Balaer, Palma de Mallorca, Spain
M Bitner-Glindzicz
Institute of Child Health, London, UK.

A Bojano
'G Rummo' Hospital, Benevento, Italy
I Borras
Ramon y Cajal Hospital, Madrid, Spain
L Boumans
University Hospital of Rotterdam, The Netherlands
U Braendle
University of Tübingen, Tübingen, Germany
KA Brown
University of Leeds, UK
HG Brunner
University Hospital of Nijmegen, The Netherlands
G Calabrese
University of Chieti, Italy
L Califano
'G Rummo' Hospital, Benevento, Italy
P Capparuccia
'G Rummo' Hospital, Benevento, Italy
GJ Carvalho
University of California San Francisco, San Francisco, California, USA
I del Castillo
Ramon y Cajal Hospital, Madrid, Spain
A Chen
University of Iowa, Iowa City, Iowa USA
A Cherechevskaia
Free University of Berlin, Germany
L Collet
Edouard Herriot Hospital, Lyon, France
A Costa
Free University of Berlin, Germany
P Coucke
University of Antwerp, Belgium
CWRJ Cremers
University Hospital of Nijmegen, The Netherlands
S Crino
University of Palermo, Italy
M Cruz Tapia
Ramon y Cajal Hospital, Madrid, Spain
O Cura
Ege University Medical School, Izmir, Turkey
B Dallapiccola
CSS Hospital, San Giovanni Rotondo, Italy
A D'Amico
University of Palermo, Italy

A Davis
MRC Institute of Hearing Research, Nottingham, UK
F Declau
University Hospital of Antwerp, Belgium
O Dias
Santa Maria Hospital, Lisbon, Portugal
RJH Ensink
University Hospital of Nijmegen, The Netherlands
B Eschen
Henkel KGaG, Düsseldorf, Germany
U Finckh-Krèmer
Free University of Berlin, Germany
H Fortnum
MRC Institute of Hearing Research, Nottingham, UK
P Franz
University of Vienna, Austria
K Fukushima
University of Iowa, Iowa City, Iowa USA
T Gelas
Edouard Herriot Hospital, Lyon, France
G Grisanti
University of Palermo, Italy
S Grisanti
Istituto Scientifico—H S Raffaele, Milano, Italy
M Gross
Free University of Berlin, Germany
JJ Han
University of California San Francisco, San Francisco, California, USA
I Hassinen
University of Oulu, Finland
SD Hatzopoulos
University of Ferrara, Italy
C Herraiz
Ramon y Cajal Hospital, Madrid, Spain
M Hess
Free University of Berlin, Germany
DM Hoover
Boys' Town National Research Hospital, Omaha, Nebraska, USA
Y IIu
New Jersey Medical School, Newark, New Jersey, USA
PM Huygen
University Hospital of Nijmegen, The Netherlands
M Iber
Ege University Medical School, Izmir, Turkey

HT Jacobs
University of Tampere, Finland
AH Janjua
University of Manchester, UK
F Javier Hernandez
Ramon y Cajal Hospital, Madrid, Spain
T Kandogan
Ege University Medical School, Izmir, Turkey
G Karban
St James's University Hospital, Leeds, UK
JB Kenyon
Boys' Town National Research Hospital, Omaha, Nebraska, USA
WJ Kimberling
Boys' Town National Research Hospital, Omaha, Nebraska, USA
L Kintrup
Henkel KGaG, Düsseldorf, Germany
H Kingma
University of Maastricht, The Netherlands
K Kirschhofer
University of Vienna, Austria
K Konradsson
University of Lund, Sweden
M Kreiss
Edouard Herriot Hospital, Lyon, France
H Kunst
University Hospital of Nijmegen, The Netherlands
AK Lalwani
University of California San Francisco, San Francisco, California, USA
SM Leal
The Rockefeller University, New York, USA
SK Lehtinen
University of Tampere, Finland
G Lina-Granade
Edouard Herriot Hospital, Lyon, France
P Lindholm
University of Oulu, Finland
M Lovett
University of Texas Southwestern Medical Center, Dallas, Texas USA
A McInerney
Institute of Child Health, London, UK
C Magarino
Hermanos Ameijeiras Hospital, Havana, Cuba
V Magnavita
University of Padua, Italy

K Majamaa
University of Oulu, Finland
E Mäki-Torkko
University of Oulu, Finland
A Mari
Tor Vergata University, Rome, Italy
B Marino
Gesu Hospital for Children and Babies, Rome, Italy
AF Markham
University of Leeds, UK
HAM Marres
University Hospital of Nijmegen, The Netherlands
E Martines
University of Palermo, Italy
A Martini
University of Ferrara, Italy
M Mazzoli
University of Ferrara, Italy
D Mändez del Castillo
Hermanos Ameijeiras Hospital, Havana, Cuba
I Menändez-Alejo
William Soler Hospital, Havana, Cuba
R Meredith .
University Hospital of Wales, Cardiff, UK
AM Meyer zum Gottesberge
Heinrich-Heine University of Düsseldorf, Germany
AN Mhatre
University of California San Francisco, San Francisco, California, USA
V Migliosi
University of Tampere, Finland
R Mingarelli
CSS Hospital San Giovanni Rotondo, Italy
A Montero
Consejeria de Sanidad del Gobiemo Balaer, Palma de Mallorca, Spain
C Morales
Sierrallana Torrelavega Hospital, Cantabria, Spain
F Moreno
Ramon y Cajal Hospital, Madrid, Spain
A Morgon
Edouard Herriot Hospital, Lyon, France
LL Moynihan
University of Leeds, UK
RF Mueller
St James's University Hospital, Leeds, UK

VE Newton
University of Manchester, UK
S Nicolis
University of Milan, Italy
G Novelli
Tor Vergata University, Rome, Italy
K O'Dell
University of Glasgow, UK
C O'Donovan
National Rehabilitation Board, Dublin, Ireland
E Orzan
University of Padua, Italy
S Ottolenghi
University of Milan, Italy
GW Padberg
University Hospital of Antwerp, Belgium
A Parving
Bispebjerg Hospital, Copenhagen, Denmark
G Parry
St Luke's Hospital, Bradford, UK
PD Phelps
The Royal National Throat, Nose and Ear Hospital, London, UK
A Pizzuti
University of Milan, Italy
A Ramesh
University of Madras, India
R Ramirez
Puerta de Hierro Hospital, Madrid, Spain
A Ratti
University of Milan, Italy
A Reuter
Karlsruhe Research Center, Germany
M Rodriguez
Ramon y Cajal Hospital, Madrid, Spain
L Romero
Ramon y Cajal Hospital, Madrid, Spain
E Rosztok
Free University of Berlin, Germany
A Rovio
University of Tampere, Finland
L Saggin
University of Padua, Italy
M Sarduy
Ramon y Cajal Hospital, Madrid, Spain

G Scarlato
University of Milan, Italy
M Schwalb
New Jersey Medical School, Newark, New Jersey, USA
ZH Shah
University of Tampere, Finland
V Silani
Maggiore Hospital, Milan, Italy
RJH Smith
University of Iowa, Iowa City, Iowa, USA
M Sorri
University of Oulu, Finland
ME Spormann-Lagodzinski
Free University of Berlin, Germany
CR Srikumari Srisailapathy
University of Madras, India
D Stephens
University Hospital of Wales, Cardiff, UK
MD Tsakanikos
P & A Kyriakou Children's Hospital, Athens, Greece
S Uimonen
University of Oulu, Finland
PH Van de Heyning
University Hospital of Antwerp, Belgium
G Van Camp
University of Antwerp, Belgium
D Van Dyck
University of Antwerp, Belgium
L Van Laer
University of Antwerp, Belgium
M Vèyrynen
University of Oulu, Finland
K Verhoeven
University Hospital of Antwerp, Belgium
M Villamar
Ramon y Cajal Hospital, Madrid, Spain
E Vitale
New Jersey Medical School, Newark, New Jersey, USA
M Waagenaar
University Hospital of Nijmegen, The Netherlands
F Wachtler
University of Vienna, Austria
S Wayne
University of Iowa, Iowa City, Iowa, USA

H Weiher
Karlsruhe Research Centre, Germany
K Weipoltshammer
University of Vienna, Austria.
K Welzl-Müller
University Clinic, Innsbruck, Austria
P Willems
University of Antwerp, Belgium
R Winter
Institute of Child Health, London, UK
FL Wuyts
University Hospital of Antwerp, Belgium
D Zanetti
University of Brescia, Italy
RIS Zbar
University of Iowa, Iowa City, Iowa, USA
HP Zenner
University of Tübingen, Tübingen, Germany
F Zhao
University Hospital of Wales, Cardiff, UK

PART I
GENE THERAPY

Chapter 1
Gene therapy for hearing disorders

AK LALWANI, GJ CARVALHO, JJ HAN and AN MHATRE

Introduction

Gene therapy is currently being used to treat many disorders, including cancer, viral infection and the degenerative and fatal diseases of the cardiovascular and the central nervous system. However, the potential use of gene therapy for alleviation of hearing impairment has not been investigated despite the absence of effective therapy for most forms of inherited hearing disorders.

The ability to introduce exogenous DNA into a cell provides the experimental basis for clinical treatment of both inherited and acquired diseases in humans via gene transfer or gene therapy (Goldspiel et al., 1993). With the rapid progress in identification of genetic factors that underlie a variety of human disease (Iannaccone and Scarpelli, 1993; Samara et al., 1993) and refinement of techniques in the introduction of these genes into mammalian cells *in vitro* and *in vivo* (Kotani et al., 1994), delivery of a 'therapeutic' gene to the patient is gaining acceptance as a viable treatment in rare as well as relatively common disorders.

Initial applications of gene therapy were focused on treatment of rare genetic disorders such as severe combined immunodeficiency disease and haemophilia (Parkman and Gelfand, 1991). Knowledge of the molecular bases of these disorders at the genetic level led to transfection of the normal version of the mutant gene into the affected tissue. The product from this transgene, stably integrated into the cellular genome, provided the functional gene product required to negate the disease phenotype. Currently, gene therapy is being used to treat many non-Mendelian disorders, including cancer (Dorudi et al., 1993), viral infection (Cournoyer and Caskey, 1993) and the degenerative and fatal diseases of the cardiovascular (French, 1993; Nabel et al., 1994) and the central nervous systems (Dunnett and Svendson, 1993). In the treatment of these disorders, the gene introduced need not be the primary cause of disorder. The criterion for selecting the therapeutic gene is that its expression, which can be transient and not limited to the affected cells or tissue, should circumvent and/or eliminate the pathology. Gene transfer has been performed successfully in a large variety of post-mitotic cells such as myotubes, hepatocytes, endothelial cells, airway epithelial cells, and a variety of neuronal cells.

An interesting target for gene therapy which has not previously been studied is the neurosensory epithelia of the inner ear. Cochlear gene therapy has experimental and therapeutic applications including facilitating the study of cochlear genes and proteins or alleviating hearing loss by the introduction of specific genes. Positional cloning studies in several large families with hereditary, non-syndromal hearing impairment will suggest potential candidate genes for gene therapy. These studies will aid in designing therapeutic strategies to alleviate auditory dysfunction as well as contributing towards molecular genetic analysis of hearing. Clinical application of gene therapy is focused towards introducing exogenous genes into somatic cells only and not into the germ line. Thus the altered genome will not be inherited.

The central issue in gene therapy is to develop methods for tissue- or cell-specific targeting of the therapeutic gene whose expression will be stable and optimally regulated. Historically, the introduction of DNA into cells has been by chemical (calcium phosphate precipitation) or physical (electroporation) methods. These are still the methods of choice for introducing DNA into cultured mammalian cells. A major disadvantage of these methods is their low efficiency. In addition, these methods do not distinguish between different cell types. Viruses that have been genetically altered so as to render them nonlytic and capable of accepting and expressing exogenous DNA represent the current choice as vectors for transfecting genes *in vivo* (Brody and Crystal, 1994). This strategy uses the highly evolved mechanism of the virus for efficient, cell-specific introduction of its genetic material in the infection process. This method involves packaging the therapeutic gene into a non-pathogenic, non-lytic virus which is then introduced into the patient, site specifically, via viral infection.

Selection of the viral vector for intracochlear gene therapy

Several viral vectors have been explored for delivery of the therapeutic gene (Cohen-Haguenauer, 1994). Each has special characteristics which make it useful in specific experimental and therapeutic paradigms. Gene therapy vectors using retrovirus, adenovirus, herpes virus and adeno-associated virus (AAV) have been tested extensively in a variety of cells.

Retroviral vectors

The prototypes for viral mediated gene transfer are the retroviruses (Williams, 1990; Merrouche and Favrot, 1992; Barba et al., 1993). Retroviral vectors are characterized by their ability only to integrate into the genome of dividing cells, and are unstable *in vivo*. Their ability to integrate selectively into dividing cells makes them the ideal vector for introducing tumoricidal factors into proliferating neoplastic cells. Neurosensory epithelia of the inner ear, being post-mitotic, are not suitable targets for retroviral vector gene transfer.

Adenoviral vectors

Adenovirus is a common human pathogen causing relatively benign syndromes, such as colds and conjunctivitis. Replication-defective adenovirus vectors are considered relatively safe (Berkener, 1992; Boviatsis et al., 1994). Unlike the retroviral vectors, the adenoviral vectors do not integrate their genes into the genome of the target cell. In addition, adenoviral vectors will infect both dividing and non-dividing cells with high efficiency and provide expression of the recombinant gene as an extra-chromosomal element for a period of only several weeks to a month. Therefore, adenoviral vectors are also hampered by temporally limited transgene expression. In addition, these vectors provoke a strong immune response which may be toxic to the recipient cell.

Herpes virus vectors

Replication-defective recombinant viruses and plasmid-derived ampli-cons are the two types of herpes virus vectors that have been developed for gene delivery into cells and tissues (Leib and Olivo, 1993; Boviatsis et al., 1994). Both types can be relatively non-pathogenic to neural tissues and can mediate transgene expression in a substantial number of neurones and other cell types. The recombinant herpes vectors have the distinct advantage that they can enter a latent state in some neuronal cells and could thus potentially mediate stable transgene expression. However, this is usually limited to a very few cells.

Adeno associated virus (AAV)

AAV is a linear single-stranded DNA parvovirus that is endogenous to many mammalian species (Muzyczka, 1992). The wild-type AAV-2 genome consists of 4680 nucleotides and contains three promoters that control genes required for replication and encapsidation of the AAV genome. For lytic growth, AAV requires coinfection with a helper virus, either adenovirus or *Herpes simplex*. When no helper virus is available, AAV can persist as an integrated provirus. When cells carrying an AAV provirus are subsequently superinfected with a helper, the integrated AAV genome is rescued and a productive lytic cycle occurs. Recent characterization of wild-type AAV integration, which requires the inverted terminal repeats, has demonstrated preferential targeting into the long arm of human chromosome 19 (Kotin et al., 1990; Samulski et al., 1991). Integration of recombinant AAV vectors lacking the *rep* gene is probably random. The ability of AAV to latently infect cells, with no apparent harm to the host, has led to investigation of AAV as a vector for gene therapy.

AAV vector for gene therapy is associated with several desirable characteristics (Muzyczka, 1992). AAV is non-pathogenic in both humans and animals and has a broad host range, including humans, monkeys, dogs and mice. AAV is able to infect and integrate into non-dividing cells with high frequency. The integration is stable and has been shown to remain in this state through 150 passages. A major disadvantage for the use of AAV is the packaging limit of 4.5 kb of foreign DNA in AAV particles, even though much of the genome is dispensable and can be replaced by genes of interest. AAV vectors have been successfully used to introduce *neo* and *gpt* marker genes, human globin genes and the cystic fibrosis transmembrane conductance regulator.

Based on the many advantages of the AAV vector, and its suitability for introducing foreign DNA into the cochlea, it was chosen for the preliminary work in injecting genes into the inner ear. Our initial goals were to establish the feasibility of gene therapy and characterize the nature of integration of foreign DNA.

Current applications of gene therapy in the cochlea

We have recently demonstrated for the first time *in vivo* expression of a foreign gene within the mammalian inner ear resulting from localized, AAV-mediated introduction (Lalwani et al., 1996). The genetic material (a β-gal reporter gene) was directly introduced into the peripheral auditory system by use of AAV as the transfection vector and Hartley guinea-pigs as the animal model. Approximately 105 particles of AAV containing the bacterial β-galactosidase (β-gal) sequence with an Ad 2 major late promoter (Figure 1.1) were infused into the cochlea of the animal with the aid of an osmotic minipump. Animals were sacrificed after two weeks. Two Hartley guinea-pigs with intracochlear saline infusion and four unoperated (non-perfused) animals served as negative control

AAV - ß-Gal Vector

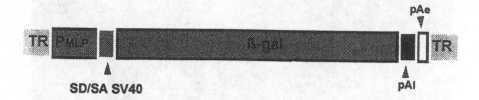

Figure 1.1 AAV-β-galactosidase vector.

subjects. Both the infused and the contralateral, non-infused cochleae were harvested from each animal, decalcified and embedded in paraffin.

Sections, 8 μm in width, were cut from the embedded cochleae and assayed for β-gal expression via immunohistochemistry. Animals perfused with AAV showed intense imunohistochemical reactivity (Figure 1.2(A)) in the spiral limbus, spiral ligament, spiral ganglion cells and the organ of Corti in the perfused cochlea and a much weaker staining but with similar pattern in the contralateral ear. Cochleae from saline-infused and unoperated animals were devoid of the DAB stain (Figure 1.2(B)).

The ability to introduce and stably express exogenous genetic material in the peripheral auditory system will have both experimental and therapeutic benefits. Experimentally, the ability to introduce genes into the inner ear will aid in understanding of the function of cochlear proteins and control of inner ear-specific genes. Therapeutically, the prompt delivery of neurotrophic factors in cases of sudden deafness or progressive hearing loss, mediated by viral vectors, could reduce the consequent tissue damage and preserve hearing. Genes identified through positional cloning studies of several large families with hereditary, progressive, non-syndromal hearing impairment represent potential targets for gene therapy. The results of this study will help to lay the groundwork for future investigations assessing the potential use of gene therapy for the alleviation of auditory dysfunction.

Acknowledgement

Funded as a pilot project of the NIH Gene Therapy Core Center Grant DK 47766 and Hearing Research Inc.

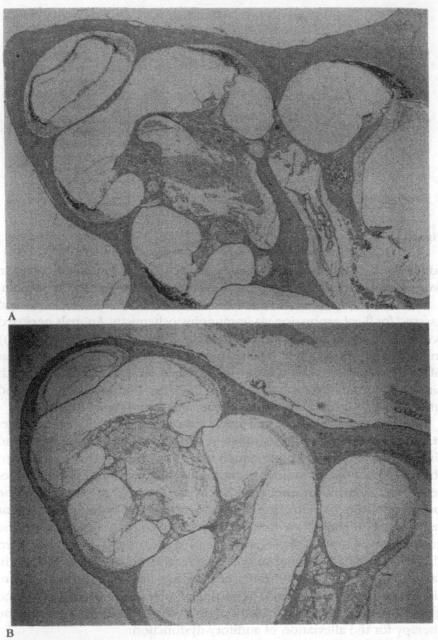

Figure 1.2 *In situ* β-gal expression within the guinea-pig cochlea. Radial sections of guinea-pig cochlea were hybridized with β-gal antibody and then developed by use of a biotin-labelled 2⁰ antibody, Vector ABC amplification system and DAB stain. (A) A radial section of the AAV-infused cochlea, extending from the base to its apex, stained for β-gal expression. Nearly all tissue types within the cochlea, including the spiral ligament, spiral limbus, the organ of Corti and the spiral ganglion, express the β-gal protein. (B) A radial section of a non-AAV-transfused cochlea, extending from the base to its apex, stained for β-gal expression. The control cochlea is devoid of the DAB stain.

PART II
RADIOLOGY

Chapter 2
Radiology of inner ear defects

PD PHELPS

Introduction

Hearing impairment from genetic abnormalities may be due to lesions of the auditory apparatus that can be demonstrated by modern imaging. Computed tomography (CT) is the standard first imaging investigation. It shows fine bone detail and the state of the middle ear which is not adequately demonstrated by magnetic resonance imaging (MRI). MRI, however, is now the imaging investigation of choice for sensorineural hearing impairment (SNHI) and can define the cranial nerves passing through the petrous temporal bone from the brainstem and also cerebrospinal fluid and the fluids of the labyrinth of the inner ear.

Results and discussion

Traditional classifications of inner ear defects are inadequate, but the following abnormalities can be identified by imaging. In order of severity with the eponym and date of original description these are:

- No inner ear (Michel, 1863).
- Primitive otocyst.
- Common cavity lesion (Cock, 1838). All are associated with anacusis and the last with a risk of a spontaneous cerebrospinal fluid fistula and/or meningitis.
- Basal cochlear gyrus and distal sac in place of the ultimate one and a half turns (Mondini, 1791; Alexander, 1904). Mondini's (1791) dissection also showed a large vestibular aqueduct (LVA) and endolymphatic sac.

7

Pendred syndrome has both Mondini cochlea and a LVA; the latter an almost constant feature (Figure 2.1).

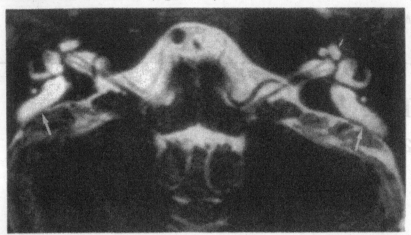

Figure 2.1 A A case of Pendred syndrome with both a Mondini cochlea and a LVA deformity. (A) An axial MRI section showing the cochlea with a reduced number of coils (small arrow) and large endolymphatic sacs (large arrow). Note the normal nerves in the IAM. (B) Sagittal section showing the same features of Mondini-type cochlea and LVA.

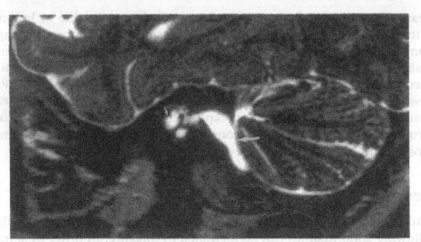

Figure 2.1 B Axial CT sections of the inner ear showing various congenital deformities.

- X-linked deformity and gusher. Bulbous internal auditory meatus (IAM) (Glasscock, 1973) and deficient bone at the fundus of the IAM (Phelps, 1991) (Figure 2.2). This characteristic deformity of the inner ear occurs in one type of X-linked deafness and seems to be associated with perilymphatic hydrops as a cerebrospinal fluid fistula only occurs if the stapes is disturbed. There is no risk of spontaneous meningitis.
- Branchio-oto-renal syndrome. Small two-turn cochlea with some skull base and middle ear deformities (Chen et al., 1995) (see Figure 2.3).

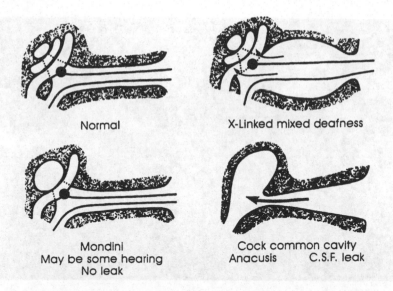

Figure 2.2 Axial CT sections of the inner ear showing various congenital deformaties.

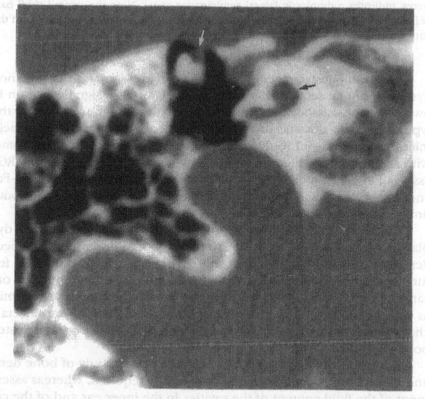

Figure 2.3 Branchio-oto-renal syndrome. Axial CT section showing a small two-turn cochlea (black arrow) and ossicular mass in the middle ear attached to the anterior wall (white arrow). A typical case of this genetic syndrome with autosomal dominant inheritance.

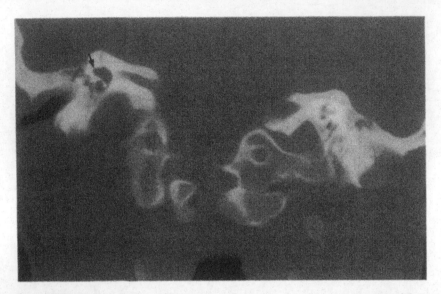

Figure 2.4. Overall skull base deformity with narrow upward-slanting IAMs shown on two coronal sections in a case of velocardiofacial (Shprintzen) syndrome. The arrow indicates a dysplastic lateral semicircular canal. Note the overall skull base deformity probably accounting for the high incidence of conductive deafness in this autosomal dominant syndrome.

The commonest congenital deformity of the labyrinth is the short dysplastic lateral semicircular canal which is of little significance on its own as it can be associated with normal cochlear function. However this type of dysplasia does occur with middle ear abnormalities in hemifacial microsomia, Treacher Collins syndrome and some other syndromes with a genetic basis (Figure 2.4). A characteristic feature of the CHARGE association is complete absence of the semicircular canals. Klippel–Feil and Wildervanck syndromes are associated with severe inner and sometimes middle ear deformities

Other hereditary abnormalties of the inner ear are the osseous dysplasias. More than 30 types of sclerosing bone dysplasias have been described (Beighton and Sellars, 1982). However, the radiological features are similar with increased density of the periosteal, but not otic capsule bone and encroachment on the canals of the petrous pyramid, as well as the middle ear cavity (Figure 2.5). Osteogenesis imperfecta is characterised by patchy rarefaction of both otic capsule and periosteal bone (Bergstrom, 1997) (see Figure 2.6).

Thus in hearing impairment of genetic origin a study of bone detail and identification of bone dysplasias by CT is required, whereas assessment of the fluid content of the cavities in the inner ear and of the cranial nerves and the brainstem is achieved by MRI.

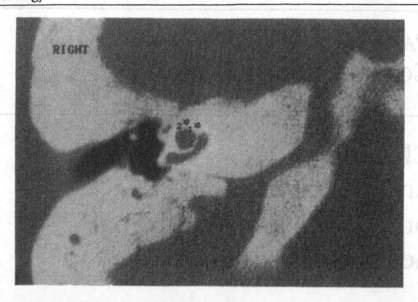

Figure 2.5 Axial CT section of the skull base in a patient with craniometaphyseal dysplasia. Densitometry readings have been taken at the otic capsule around the distal coils of the cochlea. These readings are, in fact, lower than normal but similar to the readings made at the sclerotic periosteal bone in the rest of the petrous pyramid.

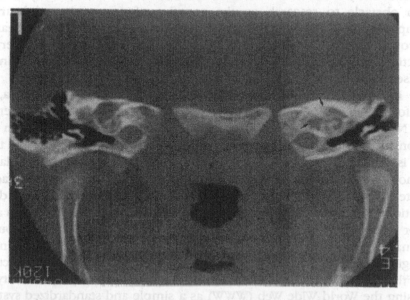

Figure 2.6 Coronal CT section in a case of osteogenesis imperfecta. Note the areas of bone rarefaction around the cochlea (arrows). Thus, in hearing impairment of genetic origin, a study of bone detail and identification of bone dysplasias by CT is required, whereas assessment of the fluid content of the cavities in the inner ear and of the cranial nerves and the brainstem is achieved by MRI.

PART III
COMPUTER SYSTEMS

Chapter 3
An Internet database on genetic non-syndromal hearing impairments

M MAZZOLI, L SAGGIN, SD HATZOPOULOS and A MARTINI

Introduction

The scarcity of affected families available in a certain area, or city is often an obstacle to research on the genetics of non-syndromal hearing impairments (NSHI). This was one of the reasons why several research groups decided to join forces and establish a European Concerted Action on Genetics of Hearing Impairment (HEAR) to coordinate research and progress in this field.

In order to circulate information and collect European-based data, an information retrieval system (IRS) from a database of families with genetic NSHI has been designed. The suggestion for a database came from the consideration that most hereditary hearing impairments are rare and that it is difficult to find affected families, especially those which are large enough to allow linkage studies. Furthermore, the database would facilitate the standardized collection of data using common terminology, definitions and testing as well as being a reference source for information and for comparison of clinical description with data from other groups. Finally, it could represent, in time, a repository of European epidemiological data. Since the use of informatics and the possibility of connecting with the Internet is increasing rapidly, we investigated the possibility of using the World Wide Web (WWW) as a simple and standardized system to make data easily available to interested users anywhere in the world.

One of the aims of the Concerted Action is to create common working platforms which are available to different groups involved in the research and the Internet seems to be the most appropriate environment to do this. In fact, other Concerted Action members have already designed Home Pages which contain information relating to research on the genetics of hearing impairment, such as the Hereditary Hearing Homepage designed at the Department of Medical Genetics of the University of Antwerp[1]. Another site may be found on the Net for collection of data about families with hereditary hearing impairment: the National Institute on Deafness and Other Communication Disorders (NIDCD) Hereditary Hearing Impairment Resource Registry[2]. In the latter a research plan is presented, but data are not accessible. For the present work it is intended to create a working platform to allow researchers to work on a common basis, although in different countries.

The IRS presented here will be linked to these and to other relevant Internet sites. It is hoped that this IRS will represent an easy-to-use tool to increase information exchange, to file data in a standardized manner, and to retrieve information for research, statistics, or clinical use, anywhere in the world.

Choice and design of software

In order to create an IRS for genetic hearing impairment the design of the database structure had to be considered in terms of field composition of the records in the database. Moreover, suitable software had to be selected in order to index the table of this database.

Database design

The important parameters that describe the clinical aspects of non-syndromal hereditary hearing impairment were utilized as fields of the records in the database, following definitions agreed upon by subgroups 1, 2 and 3 during HEAR meetings[3]. The parameters (fields) most likely to be the object of a query have been indexed with IRS software:

- Family identification code (family ID).
- Mode of inheritance.
- Range of frequencies of impairment.
- Hearing levels.
- Tinnitus.
- Type of hearing impairment.
- Type of onset.
- Progression of the impairment.
- Lateralization.
- Vestibular activity.
- Radiological malformations.
- Consanguinity.
- Ethnicity.

[1] http://dnalab-www.uia.ac.be/dnalab/hhh/index.html
[2] http://www.boystown.org/hhirr/hhirr.htm
[3] *Infoletter*, edited by European Work Group on Genetics of Hearing Impairment, Volume 2, November 1996.

Other parameters (fields) which were also included were not indexed: researcher name; institution and address; number of affected subjects; number of obligate carriers and of normal individuals and of generations studied. Furthermore, the database was designed to contain a non-indexed field whose content is a hyperlink to open graphics documents, such as the family tree. The design of this database is such that some of the parameters (fields) at present not indexed could be indexed in the future. They include, for instance, locus name and chromosome location. In addition, in the future, it will be possible to plan the additional indexing of other parameters, such as OMIM[4] number.

IRS software

In order to index this database it was decided to use software which matched the two following criteria: (a) it should be freeware; (b) it should be queried via a simple and standardized interface, such as WWW forms.

A well-known software for information retrieval, a variant of Wide Area Information Server (WAIS), called freeWAIS-sf[5], was utilized, since it presents many advantages over the original software.

In relation to the goals of this project, the most important improvements are the support for fields and for complex boolean operators. An exact definition of characters which can be indexed, freeWAIS-sf, (developed by U. Pfeifer at the University of Dortmund), is a suite of client-server programs, the most important being its indexer, waisindex. For each table and field to be indexed, freeWAIS-sf generates a series of files which can be queried by client software via a server program, part of the suite, called waisserver. The cascade of events underlying querying freeWAIS-sf indexed data via the WWW is a little complicated, and is summarized in Figure 3.1. Note that a gateway between the WWW and freeWAIS-sf was needed. This is achieved by SFgate[6], a program written in PERL[7] (by N. Goevert at the University of Dortmund). This program is especially suited for usage with freeWAIS-sf as it supports all its extensions with regard to the original WAIS. SFgate, however, is designed as a common gateway interface (CGI) script so that it is usable with any WWW server supporting the CGI standard.

SFgate is a self-contained program. For local databases, it is not even necessary to connect to waisserver; databases located on the same host as the hypertext transfer protocol (HTTP) server can be searched with the local search feature.

[4] http://www3.ncbi.nlm.n.h.gov/Omim/
[5] http://www.wsc.com/freeWAIS-sf/fwsf_toc.html
[6] http://ls6-www.informatik.uni-dortmund.de/ir/projects/SFgate/SFgate.html
[7] http://www.perl.com/perl/index.html

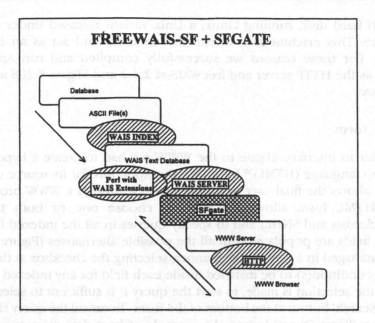

FREEWAIS-SF + SFGATE

Database

ASCII File(s)

WAIS INDEX

WAIS Text Database

Perl with
WAIS Extensions

WAIS SERVER

SFgate

WWW Server

HTTP

WWW Browser

Figure 3.1 Datasheet representing data processing from the database to a WWW browser. In short: an ASCII file containing data to be indexed is processed by waisindex and the resulting files can be searched by a WWW-based form via a WWW gateway, SFgate.

Results

Databases

Initially, two databases were designed: one describing families and the second containing specific information relative to single affected subjects, including graphic representation of clinical tests through a hyperlink to inline images. It was then agreed during the HEAR joint meeting in Milan (11–13 October 1996) to limit the information to general family data.

The 'family' database is made up of two tables: firstly, sensorineural hearing impairment (SNHI) and, secondly, otosclerosis. This subdivision of NSHI data was needed to facilitate and speed the program reply to queries for specific fields which are meaningful in some pathologies and less so in others. As mentioned above, only the fields relevant for a query were indexed. Tables filled with fictitious data to test the reliability of information retrieved by this system were created.

Setup of the server

FreeWAIS-sf and SFgate programs run only on computers based on Unix operating systems. We therefore set up an Intel Pentium 133 MHz, with a 1 Gb hard disk, running Linux, a Unix variant released under GNU license[8]. This machine had to run the database and act as an HTTP server. For these reasons we successfully compiled and run Apache 1.1.1[9] as the HTTP server and freeWAIS-sf 2.1.2 and SFgate 5.108 as IRS software.

HTML form

In order to interface SFgate to the WWW, we had to create a hypertext markup language (HTML)[10] form (see the Appendix for its source code) which allows the final user to submit queries through a WWW browser. This HTML form allows the user to choose one or both tables (Otosclerosis and SNHL) and to specify queries in all the indexed fields. These fields are populated with all the possible alternatives (Figure 3.2). All is managed in a very simple manner, selecting the checkbox at the left of the condition(s) to be matched inside each field for any indexed field. Once the selection is made, to start the query it is sufficient to select the 'Start Search' button at the bottom of the form. To cancel the query simply click on 'Reset Query' button. An example of how data are retrieved is presented in Figure 3.3. One of the fields of the record does not contain data but is a hyperlink to a graphic interexchange format (.GIF) file that reports a genetic tree for the family (see inset Figure 3.3).

A potential problem arises from the way in which SFgate (and all CGI programs) processes queries. If there is more than an input box for terms to be searched for then, from the point of view of the the boolean operator, SFgate builds the query like this:

• All the ORed terms are collected first.
• Then the ANDed terms are collected and appended to the rest of the query.

This means that queries are not processed from left to right and the answer given back could be sometimes different from what one asks for.

To solve this problem it was decided to set a hidden 'AND' to connect fields to each other while terms inside each field were connected by the logical operator 'OR'. People who want to make searches which are different from these default conditions (for example, by use of the boolean operator 'OR' instead of 'AND' between fields), can fill in a text area which is part of the HTML form.

The fine tuning of queries is also possible using an additional option at the bottom of the form. This allows the maximum number of records that can be retrieved to be changed.

[8] http://www.linux.org/
[9] http://www.apache.org/
[10] http://www/utoronto.ca/webdocs/HTMLdocs/NewHTML/html_intro.html

Select one or both of these databases:

☑ SNHL
☑ Otosclerosis

Enter your query conditions:

MODE OF INHERITANCE
☑ Autosomal Dominant   ☐ X-linked Dominant   ☐ Polygenic
☐ Autosomal Recessive   ☐ X-linked Recessive   ☐ Unknown
☐ Mitochondrial

RANGE OF FREQUENCY IMPAIRMENT
☑ Low   ☐ High   ☐ Mid+High   ☐ Extended High
☐ Mid   ☐ Low+Mid   ☐ Low+High   ☐ All Frequencies

Low: < 500Hz   High: > 2000Hz and =< 8000Hz
Mid: 500 - 2000Hz   Extended High: > 8000Hz

HEARING LEVELS
☑ Mild   ☐ Moderate   ☐ Severe   ☐ Profound

Mild: < 40dB   Severe: 70 - 94dB
Moderate: 40 - 69dB   Profound: >= 95dB
Average across 500, 1000, 2000 and 4000Hz (PTA) of the better hearing ear

HEARING IMPAIRMENT TYPE
☐ Conductive   ☐ Mixed   ☐ Sensorineural

TYPE OF ONSET
☐ Congenital   ☐ Late   ☐ Uncertain

PROGRESSION
☐ Stable   ☐ Progressive

LATERALIZATION
☐ Bilateral   ☐ Unilateral

VESTIBULAR INVOLVEMENT
☐ Involved   ☐ Uninvolved   ☐ Uncertain

CONSANGUINITY
☐ Present   ☐ Absent   ☐ Uncertain

For Experts Only:

| Start Search | | Reset Query |

Additional options:

1. How many hits do you want at most? 30
   You can specify how many hit you want at most (they must be between 1 and 99).

THIS PAGE REFERENCES:
© 1995-96 BioPD - University of Padova - Author Leopoldo Saggin
Mail to: lsaggin@civ.bio.unipd.it - Last Revision: October 1, 1996 - Tested on Netscape 1.2
Best viewed on Netscape 2.0 or higher

Figure 3.2. The query form as it appears connecting at: http://hear.unife.it/ audiology. Each field contains all possible choices and were identified according to terminology definitions published in *Infoletter 2*. Selection of the details of the query is easily done by selecting the checkbox on the left side of the term, as seen in this example.

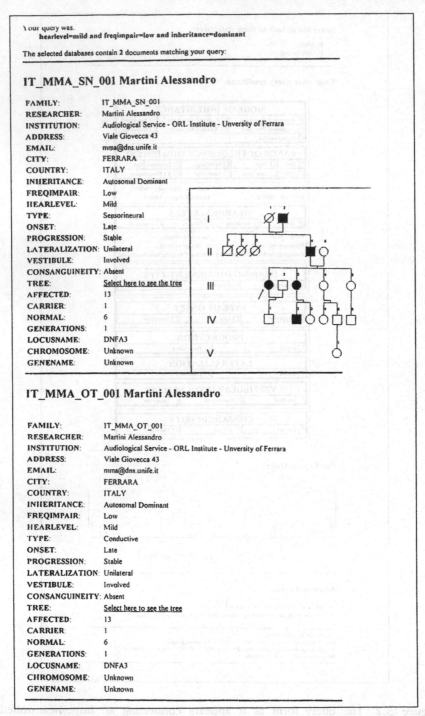

Your query was.
    hearlevel=mild and freqimpair=low and inheritance=dominant

The selected databases contain 2 documents matching your query:

IT_MMA_SN_001 Martini Alessandro

FAMILY:	IT_MMA_SN_001
RESEARCHER:	Martini Alessandro
INSTITUTION:	Audiological Service - ORL Institute - Unversity of Ferrara
ADDRESS:	Viale Giovecca 43
EMAIL:	mma@dns.unife.it
CITY:	FERRARA
COUNTRY:	ITALY
INHERITANCE:	Autosomal Dominant
FREQIMPAIR:	Low
HEARLEVEL:	Mild
TYPE:	Sensorineural
ONSET:	Late
PROGRESSION:	Stable
LATERALIZATION:	Unilateral
VESTIBULE:	Involved
CONSANGUINEITY:	Absent
TREE:	Select here to see the tree
AFFECTED:	13
CARRIER:	1
NORMAL:	6
GENERATIONS:	1
LOCUSNAME:	DNFA3
CHROMOSOME:	Unknown
GENENAME:	Unknown

IT_MMA_OT_001 Martini Alessandro

FAMILY:	IT_MMA_OT_001
RESEARCHER:	Martini Alessandro
INSTITUTION:	Audiological Service - ORL Institute - Unversity of Ferrara
ADDRESS:	Viale Giovecca 43
EMAIL:	mma@dns.unife.it
CITY:	FERRARA
COUNTRY:	ITALY
INHERITANCE:	Autosomal Dominant
FREQIMPAIR:	Low
HEARLEVEL:	Mild
TYPE:	Conductive
ONSET:	Late
PROGRESSION:	Stable
LATERALIZATION:	Unilateral
VESTIBULE:	Involved
CONSANGUINEITY:	Absent
TREE:	Select here to see the tree
AFFECTED:	13
CARRIER:	1
NORMAL:	6
GENERATIONS:	1
LOCUSNAME:	DNFA3
CHROMOSOME:	Unknown
GENENAME:	Unknown

Figure 3.3 Example of data retrieved with the choices made in Figure 3.2. Note that the underlined field is a hyperlink to the .GIF image representing the family tree, as shown in the inset. Note also that data are not real but fictitious, for testing the database reliability.

This query form and the related database was made accessible to anyone accessing the database web page, while sending data by use of a login and a password, so it has limited sharing, i.e. to HEAR members only.

Discussion

This paper reports the design of an IRS with data relative to families affected by NSHI. Initially, two databases were designed: one describing families and the second containing specific information relative to single affected subjects, including graphic representation of clinical tests through a hyperlink to inline images. At the HEAR joint meeting in Milan (11–13 October 1996) it was agreed to limit the information to the general family data, whereas a second database, linked to the family database, should contain phenotypic descriptions.
It was decided to use an IRS because:

- There are many reliable information retrieval packages which may be downloaded (free of charge) from the Net and a free database engine is still lacking.
- IRS reduces the possibility of human error in loading data to the database, since data input relies on one or a few people.

The aim of this project is, however, the evolution from an IRS to a true database, i.e. a system whereby each user cannot only search data but can also input or modify their own contributed data. Such a system presents the advantage of having the information 'on-line'. In this case one of the main problems to solve when designing the database is to guarantee the security of data so that information cannot be modified by users other than the researcher who originally presented the information.
Another problem is the choice of the database engine. At present, there is much effort aimed at the development of free database engines which may be searched through the WWW and the definition of some standards is likely in a very short time.

Conclusions

The scarcity of affected families available in a certain area, or city is often an obstacle to research on genetics of NSHI. In order to circulate information and collect European-based data, an IRS from a database of families with genetic NSHI has been designed. Since the use of informatics and the possibility of connecting to the Internet is increasing rapidly, a WWW query form was created to make data easily available to interested users anywhere in the world.
The database was indexed by use of a WAIS derivative, freeWAIS-sf. To make this indexed data available in the WWW environment a CGI, writ-

ten in PERL and called SFgate, has been used. The database is accessible by use of a password and may have limited sharing.

This retrieval system could represent an easy-to-use tool to increase information exchange, to file data in a standardized manner and to retrieve information for research, statistics and clinical use, anywhere in the world.

Appendix I
Source code of the HTML

```
<HTML>
<HEAD>
<TITLE>Hearing Impairment: Family Database</TITLE>
</HEAD>
<BODY BACKGROUND="audiobkg.gif">
<FORM METHOD=POST ACTION="/htbin/SFgate">
<CENTER>
<A
HREF="http://wwwfog.bio.unipd.it/cgibin/imagemap/audiology/family1.map">
<IMG SRC="../gif/fam_bar1.gif" ISMAP></A>
</CENTER>
<PRE>

</PRE>

<H2>Select one or both of these databases:</H2>
<DL>
<DD><INPUT NAME="database" TYPE="checkbox"
    VALUE="local//wais-sources/audiology/snhl">
<FONT SIZE=+1><B>SNHL</B></FONT>
<DD><INPUT NAME="database" TYPE="checkbox"
    VALUE="local//wais-sources/audiology/otosclrs">
<FONT SIZE=+1><B>Otosclerosis</B></FONT>
</DL>
<P>
<HR>

<H2>Enter your query conditions:</H2>

<CENTER>

<TABLE BORDER>
<TR><TH> </TH><TH>
<TABLE BORDER WIDTH="100%">
<TR><TH ALIGN=center COLSPAN=3><FONT SIZE=+2>MODE OF
    INHERITANCE</FONT></TH></TR>
<TR><TH ALIGN=left><INPUT TYPE="checkbox" NAME="inheritance_content"
    VALUE="dominant"> Autosomal Dominant</TD>
  <TH ALIGN=left><INPUT TYPE="checkbox" NAME="inheritance_content"
    VALUE="x-linked_dominant"> X-linked Dominant</TD>
  <TH ALIGN=left><INPUT TYPE="checkbox"
    NAME="inheritance_content" VALUE="polygenic"> Polygenic</TD></TR>
<TR><TH ALIGN=left><INPUT TYPE="checkbox" NAME="inheritance_content"
```

```
    VALUE="recessive"> Autosomal Recessive</TD>
  <TH ALIGN=left><INPUT TYPE="checkbox" NAME="inheritance_content"
   VALUE="x-linked_recessive"> X-linked Recessive</TD>
  <TH ALIGN=left><INPUT TYPE="checkbox" NAME="inheritance_content"
   VALUE="unknown"> Unknown</TD></TR>
<TR><TH ALIGN=left><INPUT TYPE="checkbox" NAME="inheritance_content"
   VALUE="mitochondrial"> Mitochondrial</TD></TR>
</TABLE>

</TH></TR>
<TR><TD> </TD></TR>
<TR><TH> </TH><TH>

<TABLE BORDER WIDTH="100%">
<TR><TH ALIGN=center COLSPAN=4><FONT SIZE=+2>RANGE OF FREQUENCY
   IMPAIRMENT</FONT></TH></TR>
<TR><TH ALIGN=left><INPUT TYPE="checkbox" NAME="freqimpair_content"
   VALUE="low"> Low</TD>
  <TH ALIGN=left><INPUT TYPE="checkbox" NAME="freqimpair_content"
   VALUE="high"> High</TD>
  <TH ALIGN=left><INPUT TYPE="checkbox" NAME="freqimpair_content"
   VALUE="mid+high"> Mid+High</TD>
  <TH ALIGN=left><INPUT TYPE="checkbox" NAME="freqimpair_content"
   VALUE="extended_high"> Extended High</TD></TR>

<TR><TH ALIGN=left><INPUT TYPE="checkbox" NAME="freqimpair_content"
   VALUE="mid"> Mid</TD>
  <TH ALIGN=left><INPUT TYPE="checkbox" NAME="freqimpair_content"
   VALUE="low+mid"> Low+Mid</TD>
  <TH ALIGN=left><INPUT TYPE="checkbox" NAME="freqimpair_content"
   VALUE="low+high"> Low+High</TD>
  <TH ALIGN=left><INPUT TYPE="checkbox" NAME="freqimpair_content"
   VALUE="frequencies"> All Frequencies</TD></TR>
</TABLE>

</TH></TR>
<TR><TD> </TD></TR>
<TR><TH> </TH><TH>

<TABLE WIDTH="100%">
<TR><TD WIDTH=50%><B>Low:</B> &lt; 500Hz</TD><TD><B>High:</B> &gt; 2000Hz
   and =&lt; 8000Hz</TD></TR>
<TR><TD WIDTH=50%><B>Mid:</B> 500 - 2000Hz</TD><TD><B>Extended High:</B>
   &gt; 8000Hz </TD></TR>
</TABLE>
```

```
</TH></TR>
<TR><TD> </TD></TR>
<TR><TH> </TH><TH>

<TABLE BORDER WIDTH="100%">
<TR><TH ALIGN=center COLSPAN=4><FONT SIZE=+2>
    HEARING LEVELS</FONT></TH></TR>
<TR><TH WIDTH=25% ALIGN=left><INPUT TYPE="checkbox"
    NAME="hearlevel_content" VALUE="mild"> Mild</TD>
  <TH WIDTH=25% ALIGN=left><INPUT TYPE="checkbox"
    NAME="hearlevel_content" VALUE="moderate"> Moderate</TD>
  <TH WIDTH=25% ALIGN=left><INPUT TYPE="checkbox"
    NAME="hearlevel_content" VALUE="severe"> Severe</TD>
  <TH WIDTH=25% ALIGN=left><INPUT TYPE="checkbox"
    NAME="hearlevel_content" VALUE="profound"> Profound</TD></TR>
</TABLE>

</TH></TR>
<TR><TD> </TD></TR>
<TR><TH> </TH><TH>

<TABLE WIDTH="100%">
<TR><TD WIDTH=50%><B>Mild:</B> &lt; 40dB</TD><TD><B>Severe:</B> 70 -
94dB</TD></TR>
<TR><TD WIDTH=50%><B>Moderate:</B> 40 - 69dB</TD><TD><B>Profound:</B>
&gt;=
95dB</TD></TR>
<TR><TD COLSPAN=2>Average across 500, 1000, 2000 and 4000Hz (PTA) of the
better hearing ear</TD><TR>
</TABLE>

</TH></TR>
<TR><TD> </TD></TR>
<TR><TH> </TH><TH>

<TABLE BORDER WIDTH="100%">
<TR><TH ALIGN=center COLSPAN=3><FONT SIZE=+2>HEARING IMPAIRMENT
    TYPE</FONT></TH></TR>
<TR><TH WIDTH=34% ALIGN=left><INPUT TYPE="checkbox" NAME="type_content"
    VALUE="conductive"> Conductive</TD>
  <TH WIDTH=33% ALIGN=left><INPUT TYPE="checkbox" NAME="type_content"
    VALUE="mixed"> Mixed</TD>
  <TH WIDTH=33% ALIGN=left><INPUT TYPE="checkbox" NAME="type_content"
    VALUE="sensorineural"> Sensorineural</TD></TR>
</TABLE>
```

```
</TH></TR>
<TR><TD> </TD></TR>
<TR><TH> </TH><TH>


<TABLE BORDER WIDTH="100%">
<TR><TH ALIGN=center COLSPAN=3><FONT SIZE=+2>TYPE OF
    ONSET</FONT></TH></TR>
<TR><TH WIDTH=34% ALIGN=left><INPUT TYPE="checkbox" NAME="onset_content"
  VALUE="congenital"> Congenital</TD>
  <TH WIDTH=33% ALIGN=left><INPUT TYPE="checkbox" NAME="onset_content"
  VALUE="late"> Late</TD>
  <TH WIDTH=33% ALIGN=left><INPUT TYPE="checkbox" NAME="onset_content"
  VALUE="uncertain"> Uncertain</TD></TR>
</TABLE>

</TH></TR>
<TR><TD> </TD></TR>
<TR><TH> </TH><TH>


<TABLE BORDER WIDTH="100%">
<TR><TH ALIGN=center COLSPAN=2><FONT SIZE=+2>PROGRESSION</FONT></TH></TR>
<TR><TH WIDTH=50% ALIGN=left><INPUT TYPE="checkbox"
   NAME="progression_content" VALUE="stable"> Stable</TD>
  <TH WIDTH=50% ALIGN=left><INPUT TYPE="checkbox"
   NAME="progression_content" VALUE="progressive">
   Progressive</TD></TR>
</TABLE>

</TH></TR>
<TR><TD> </TD></TR>
<TR><TH> </TH><TH>


<TABLE BORDER WIDTH="100%">
<TR><TH ALIGN=center COLSPAN=2><FONT SIZE=+2>
   LATERALIZATION</FONT></TH></TR>
<TR><TH WIDTH=50% ALIGN=left><INPUT TYPE="checkbox"
  NAME="lateralization_content" VALUE="bilateral"> Bilateral</TD>
  <TH WIDTH=50% ALIGN=left><INPUT TYPE="checkbox"
  NAME="lateralization_content" VALUE="unilateral"> Unilateral</TD></TR>
</TABLE>

</TH></TR>
<TR><TD> </TD></TR>
<TR><TH> </TH><TH>


<TABLE BORDER WIDTH="100%">
<TR><TH ALIGN=center COLSPAN=3><FONT SIZE=+2>VESTIBULAR
```

```
        INVOLVEMENT</FONT></TH></TR>
<TR><TH WIDTH=34% ALIGN=left><INPUT TYPE="checkbox"
    NAME="vestibule_content" VALUE="involved"> Involved</TD>
    <TH WIDTH=33% ALIGN=left><INPUT TYPE="checkbox"
    NAME="vestibule_content" VALUE="uninvolved"> Uninvolved</TD>
    <TH WIDTH=33% ALIGN=left><INPUT TYPE="checkbox"
    NAME="vestibule_content" VALUE="uncertain"> Uncertain</TD></TR>
</TABLE>


</TH></TR>
<TR><TD> </TD></TR>
<TR><TH> </TH><TH>

<TABLE BORDER WIDTH="100%">
<TR><TH align=center COLSPAN=3>
    <FONT SIZE=+2>CONSANGUINEITY</FONT></TH></TR>
<TR><TH WIDTH=34% ALIGN=left><INPUT TYPE="checkbox"
    NAME="consanguineity_content" VALUE="present"> Present</TD>
    <TH WIDTH=33% ALIGN=left><INPUT TYPE="checkbox"
    NAME="consanguineity_content" VALUE="absent"> Absent</TD>
    <TH WIDTH=33% ALIGN=left><INPUT TYPE="checkbox"
    NAME="consanguineity_content" VALUE="uncertain"> Uncertain</TD></TR>
</TABLE>


</TH></TR>
</TABLE>

</CENTER>
<P>
<HR>
<H2>For Experts Only:</H2>
<CENTER>
<TEXTAREA NAME="text" ROWS=3 COLS=60></TEXTAREA>
</CENTER>
<P>
<HR>
<P>


<CENTER>
<TABLE>
<TR><TH><INPUT TYPE="submit" VALUE="Start Search"></TH>
<TH> </TH>
<TH><INPUT TYPE="reset" VALUE="Reset Query"></TH></TR>
</TABLE>
</CENTER>
<P>
<HR>
<P>
```

```
<H2>Additional options:</H2>
<P>
<INPUT TYPE="hidden" NAME="tie" VALUE="and">
<INPUT TYPE="hidden" NAME="application" VALUE="family">
<INPUT TYPE="hidden" NAME="tieinternal" VALUE="or">
<INPUT TYPE="hidden" NAME="listenv" VALUE="table">
<INPUT TYPE="hidden" NAME="range" VALUE="1">
<INPUT TYPE="hidden" NAME="convert" VALUE="Table">


<OL>
<LI><B>How many hits do you want at most?</B>
 <INPUT NAME="maxhits" TYPE=TEXT VALUE="30" SIZE=2 MAXLENGTH=2>
<DL>
<DT>You can specify how many hit you want at most (they must be between
<B>1</B> and <B>99</B>).<P> </DL>
</OL>
</FORM>
<P>
<HR>
THIS PAGE REFERENCES:<BR>&#169; 1995-96
<a href="http://www.bio.unipd.it/">BioPD</a> - University of Padova -
Author: <a href="http://www.bio.unipd.it/people/leopoldo.html">
Leopoldo Saggin</a><BR>
Mail to:
<A HREF="mailto:lsaggin@civ.bio.unipd.it">lsaggin@civ.bio.unipd.it</A> -
Last Revision: <I>October 1, 1996</I> - Tested on <I>Netscape
1.22</I>.<BR>
Best viewed on <I>Netscape 2.0</I> or higher<hr>
</BODY>
</HTML>
```

Chapter 4
A decision support system for the diagnosis of syndromal genetic hearing impairment

S CRINO, A D'AMICO, S GRISANTI and G GRISANTI

The clinical problem

'In the last 20 years, many epidemiological studies have shown an increased number of cases affected by genetic hearing impairment, ranging between 9–46% of all the causes of hearing impairment with a prevalence estimate of 88:100 000 children, minimum' (European Working Group on Genetics of Hearing Impairment, 23–24 September 1994).

In the past, several authors (Anderson and Wedenberg, 1968; Konigsmark and Gorlin, 1976; Paparella, 1985) have argued that about 50% of profound childhood hearing impairments have a genetic aetiology although most of them are classified as 'of unknown origin', because of the difficulties encountered when formulating the diagnosis.

In addition, about 70% of children with genetic hearing impairments have recessive inheritance in which the parents will be clinically normal but are carriers of the trait. These cases are the most difficult to diagnose because the anamnestic data do not provide any clues.

About 30–35% of all children with genetic hearing impairment have more complex syndromes whose phenotypes are characterized by different alterations in several organs and systems (ears, eyes, genitourinary, cardiovascular, respiratory, digestive, musculoskeletal, nervous and endocrine systems). These organs and systems can be involved singly or are associated in different combinations. The organ most often involved in genetic syndromes with hearing impairment is the eye, comprising 42% of cases (Gorlin et al., 1995), which is also confirmed in our own experience (Grisanti et al., 1992).

In the literature, about 350 syndromes with different phenotypes and genotypes associated with hearing impairment have been described. The phenotypes are often not specific for a single syndrome, but are usually shared by many different syndromes, confusing the diagnosis (Ruben et al., 1991; Winter and Baraitser, 1993; Gorlin et al., 1995; Strachan and Read, 1995). The immediate phenotypic diagnosis of a syndromal hearing impairment is very difficult because:

• These syndromes are extremely polymorphous and numerous.
• Very few cases have been reported.
• A great number of clinical signs must be investigated to identify a single phenotype.

Therefore, an accurate diagnosis is essential for genetic counselling.

Fisch (1981) commented, 'The discovery of the connection between the defective hearing system and other disorders, can lead to a better understanding of causation of deafness'.

In this context, computer-based expert systems (ES) can provide a powerful tool for improving the accuracy of diagnosis of rare genetic syndromes (Grisanti et al., 1996).

G-DEAFNEX

An expert system (ES) is a software tool used to resolve complex problems which otherwise would require extraordinary knowledge and capability in the field. These complex problems are solved by simulating the human diagnostic reasoning process by use of specific knowledge and inferences (Rolston, 1988).

G-DEAFNEX (Genetic DEAFNess EXpert system) is an ES supporting the phenotypic diagnosis of syndromal genetic hearing impairment (D'Amico et al., 1993).

There is a substantial difference between a database and an ES. Databases are files containing numbers and coded data, i.e. they are systems that can only memorize information and provide it when requested. An ES can emulate the means of reasoning of a human expert. An ES is implemented through specific software elaborated by an expert in artificial intelligence (a 'knowledge engineer') with the collaboration of the expert in the field of application, in this case a physician.

Depending on the clinical signs which are inserted by the system user, G-DEAFNEX activates a series of rules that lead to the identification of the most likely syndrome or syndromes. In G-DEAFNEX about 250 syndromes with hearing impairment are represented. The ES examines over 400 non-auditory clinical signs, involving a variety of organs and systems that can be associated with the hearing impairment. The different possible combinations permit the phenotypic diagnosis of syndromic genetic hearing impairment. The ES also contains an explanation program which provides information about the syndromes and diagnostic procedure.

Input interface

G-DEAFNEX receives data relative to the hearing impairment character-istics, information about the organs and systems involved in the syn-drome and the clinical signs presented by the patient through 18 'input cards'. The first card (opening card), summarizes all the organs and sys-tems that may be involved in the syndromes contained in the ES (Figure 4.1). The other 17 cards contain all the clinical signs referring to the var-ious organs and systems which the user can indicate as 'present', 'absent' or 'don't know' (Figure 4.2).

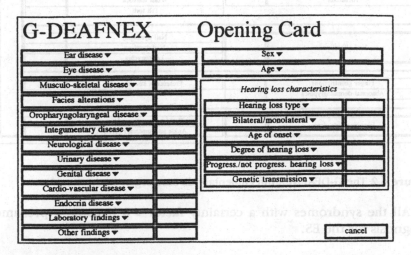

Figure 4.1 The G-DEAFNEX opening card.

Knowledge base

In G-DEAFNEX's knowledge base, the relationship between clinical signs and syndromes is represented by 'production rules':

$$\text{IF (condition) ... THEN (conclusion)}$$

The rules generally increase or decrease opportune 'certainty factors' (CF) (Shortliffe, 1976), one for any syndrome. Each rule is independent of the others and, in general, the rules can be activated in any order. There are three groups of rules:

- Organ or system rules (OR): evaluate the user's indications of the organs and systems involved in a syndrome.
- Sign rules (SR): evaluate the user's indications of the clinical signs present in the patient.
- Medical knowledge rules (MR): express medical expertise.

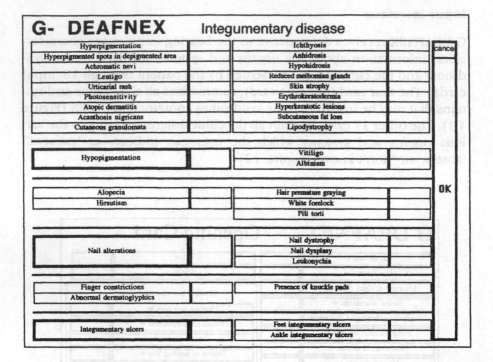

Figure 4.2 The G-DEAFNEX integumentary disease organ card.

All the syndromes with a certainty factor >0 become a presumed diagnosis for the ES.

System architecture

The diagnostic procedure may be viewed as a loop. The first part represents the 'diagnostic hypotheses', followed by 'the request for special tests that confirm or exclude the initial hypotheses' and the last part has the 'final diagnostic hypotheses'. Each time a complete loop is performed, the number of diagnostic hypotheses is reduced.

Stefanelli (1988) formalized the diagnostic process in abduction, deduction and induction phases (Figure 4.3).

The elementary cognitive processes of abduction, deduction and induction are utilized by G-DEAFNEX, with eventual repetitions, in its reasoning process. The degree of certainty of the proposed diagnosis by G-DEAFNEX, reflects the amount and consistency of the data that verify it. G-DEAFNEX's architecture is the following:

- Abduction phase: G-DEAFNEX begins by examining the data regarding the organs and systems involved in the syndrome that are provided as input. In this phase the ORs operate.

- Deductive phase: G-DEAFNEX begins its deductive phase with the candidate syndromes obtained in the previous phase. The ES narrows down these syndromes by asking the user if the clinical signs specific for those syndromes are present in the patient.
- Inductive phase: if in the previous phase further input was provided, the ES, utilizing the MRs and the SRs, begins the elimination inductive phase. In this phase, all the syndromes that have their necessary clinical signs indicated by the user as absent or that have a different type of hearing impairment (relative to the specific syndrome being considered) are excluded. After this phase the ES provides its output.

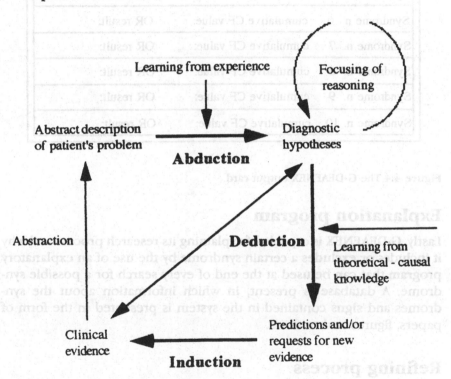

Figure 4.3 Epistemological model of diagnostic reasoning (Stefanelli, 1988).

Output interface

G-DEAFNEX uses a very simple card to suggest the proposed diagnosis. On this card the ES lists the syndromes which are candidates for diagnoses and the OR's results for these syndromes. It lists these candidate diagnoses in order of decreasing cumulative CF values (Figure 4.4).

G-DEAFNEX	Proposed diagnoses	
Syndrome n. 1	cumulative CF value:	OR result:
Syndrome n. 2	cumulative CF value:	OR result:
Syndrome n. 3	cumulative CF value:	OR result:
Syndrome n. 4	cumulative CF value:	OR result:
Syndrome n. 5	cumulative CF value:	OR result:
Syndrome n. 6	cumulative CF value:	OR result:
Syndrome n. 7	cumulative CF value:	OR result:
Syndrome n. 8	cumulative CF value:	OR result:
Syndrome n. 9	cumulative CF value:	OR result:
Syndrome n. 10	cumulative CF value:	OR result:

Figure 4.4 The G-DEAFNEX output card.

Explanation program

Lastly, G-DEAFNEX is capable of explaining its research process and why it includes or excludes a certain syndrome by the use of an explanatory program that can be used at the end of every search for a possible syndrome. A database is present, in which information about the syndromes and signs contained in the system is presented in the form of papers, figures and outlines.

Refining process

Three groups of data and several validation steps were used to refine G-DEAFNEX. These three data groups include, respectively:

- Patients with a known diagnosis.
- Simulation of cases by human experts.
- Research references used to simulate extremely rare syndromes.

Technical data and implementation

G-DEAFNEX is implemented on a Power Macintosh computer, and needs at least 16 Mb of RAM to operate. The computation time required to complete one diagnostic cycle is between 3–10 min depending on the data given as input by the user and on the number of requests for new data that the ES makes.

The ES can accept any further addition of new syndromes and clinical signs in the knowledge base.

Discussion

The diagnosis of a genetic hearing impairment is very important when planning the therapy and rehabilitation of the patient, forecasting the prognosis, evaluating the risk of transmitting the condition to eventual offspring and for genetic counselling. The ultimate goal of the present work is to provide the physicians with a useful tool to rapidly and accurately identify hearing impairments associated with rare genetic syndromes.

Apart from the audiological point of view, there is clear evidence that computer-based ESs can enhance our knowledge in rapidly growing areas of biomedical sciences. Improved diagnostic tools can support studies of gene identification and cloning by providing larger cohorts of patients. Gene identification represents the necessary background for gene therapy technology which could be applied to the treatment of hearing impairments associated with genetic syndromal/non-syndromal diseases without effective therapy. A great number of technical difficulties must be solved before gene replacement can be considered a feasible therapeutical approach in humans. Recently, Lalwani et al. (1996) reported the successful application of a viral mediated gene transfer technique to the auditory system of Hartley guinea-pigs. In that study direct intracochlear infusion of viral vectors resulted in stable integration and expression of the marker gene into neuroepithelial cells of the inner ear and contiguous tissues.

A better comprehension of genetic syndromes with hearing impairment in combination with molecular biology techniques will open up new possibilities in terms of the diagnostic and therapeutic approaches and will contribute to the elimination or at least alleviation of auditory symptoms in affected patients.

Conclusion

The value of G-DEAFNEX as an aid in the diagnosis of genetic syndromes with hearing impairment is evident. It not only offers a 'presumptive' diagnosis, but it also serves as a study aid, providing a list of clinical signs which might otherwise have been overlooked and which stimulate thought. If the user has any questions about the clinical signs, the database contained in G-DEAFNEX provides a definition or brief description of all the clinical signs. Often these seemingly insignificant clinical signs are crucial for the correct diagnosis of very rare genetic syndromes with hearing impairment.

Last, but not least, G-DEAFNEX has an 'explanation system', which is capable of explaining why a syndrome was considered as the presumed diagnosis and why another syndrome was not.

Physicians occasionally encounter patients in whom the hearing impairment is associated with a variety of clinical signs. In these cases they may suspect a genetic syndrome but, usually due to the complexity of determining which genetic syndrome it is, they are seldom able to specify the syndrome.

G-DEAFNEX is an aid to the diagnosis of genetic syndromes with hearing impairment. The techniques and methods of artificial intelligence were applied to develop this expert system.

G-DEAFNEX, using many different software 'production rules' provides the presumed diagnosis.

The various procedures that G-DEAFNEX uses to provide the 'presumptive diagnosis' have been described in the text.

Acknowledgements

The study was supported by grants from the Italian Ministero dell'Università e della Ricerca Scientifica e Tecnologica.

PART IV
EPIDEMIOLOGY

Chapter 5
Epidemiology of hereditary hearing impairment in childhood — preliminary estimates from the European Union

A PARVING, RJC ADMIRAAL, F APAYDIN, E ARSLAN, A DAVIS,
O DIAS, H FORTNUM, G GRISANTI, M GROSS, M HESS,
K KONRADSSON, G LINA-GRANADE, E MÄKI-TORKKO,
VE NEWTON, C O'DONOVAN, E ORZAN, M SORRI,
D STEPHENS, MD TSAKANIKOS, M WAAGENAAR and
K WELZL-MÜLLER

Introduction

In a previous EEC survey, comprising the 1969 birth cohort, an estimated prevalence of 0.9/1000 children with hearing impairment $\geqslant$50 dB HL for the better hearing ear, averaged across 0.5–4 kHz was found with a proportion of 9% ascribed to heredity (Martin et al., 1981). In more recent studies from various countries and local areas in Europe, a proportion of 30–50% of hereditary hearing impairment has been indicated (for a review see Parving, 1996). However, due to differences in hearing levels and lack of defined cohorts, no comparisons or aggregation of data could be performed. Thus, as part of the EU Concerted Action: (EU-CA) on Genetics and Hearing Impairment, the Working Group on Epidemiology has performed a survey of hereditary hearing impairment from various areas. This contribution describes the preliminary data, including prevalence estimates, in terms of numbers and proportions of genetic factors causing hearing impairment.

Procedure

A questionnaire (see the Appendix) was distributed to key people in various European countries, who had data and expressed an interest in participating in the survey. From the questionnaire it appeared that all the respondents ($N=12$), representing information from 18 different nations and/or local areas, had access to clinical samples. In addition, many had access to data in schools for the deaf and hearing disabled, and follow-up from screening, whereas only four had data based on population studies.

A categorization of the factors causing hearing impairment reported for the birth cohorts 1975–1979 was used (Parving et al., 1996). From the questionnaire it appeared that most data were available for more recent birth cohorts. However, to avoid the well-known problems associated with an under-ascertainment of hearing-impaired children, it was decided to concentrate on the birth cohorts 1985–1989.

A preliminary survey of the proportions of different causative factors demonstrated some inconsistencies in the criteria for diagnosing a hereditary hearing impairment. In order to obtain an estimate as appropriate as possible of hereditary hearing impairment, consensus on the criteria was obtained, and the preliminary data were revised. Consequently, the present reported preliminary results on the prevalence of hereditary hearing impairment are based on identical birth cohorts, hearing level, and uniform criteria for inheritance based on: family history i.e.

* One or both parents/grandparents affected,
  – two or more generations affected,
  – pedigree suggesting inheritance,
  – two or more children with unaffected parents,
  – consanguinity to any degree;
  – only child with unaffected parents but with affected cousin(s);
  or
* pedigree indicating X-linked inheritance;
* pedigree indicating mitochondrial inheritance;
* recognized syndrome.

Results

Prevalence of hearing impairment

Table 5.1 demonstrates the estimated prevalence of hearing impairment as indicated in the questionnaires. The data are predominantly based on local estimates, and only the prevalences from Wales and Denmark are based on national data. Due to varying criteria for hearing impairment, differences in cohorts and insufficient demographic statistics no aggregation of, or comparison between the estimated prevalences can be performed. Future uniform criteria and definitions will result in revisions of the estimated prevalences in Table 5.1.

Table 5.1 Estimated prevalence of childhood hearing impairment per thousand live births in children born 1975–1979

Countries/areas	Prevalence
Austria	0.8
Denmark	1.3
England	1.2–4.2
Finland	0.8–1.2
France	No data available
Germany	No data available
Ireland	1.3
Italy (Sicily)	2.3
The Netherlands	No data available
Portugal	No data available
Sweden	1.1
Wales	0.8

Factors causing hearing impairment

Table 5.2 shows the proportion of hereditary hearing impairment (i.e. BEHL 0.5-4 kHz ≥50 dB) in the birth cohorts 1985–1989 from some local areas in various European countries. Most of the samples are small, precluding valid comparisons. However, as the data are based on uniform definitions and criteria, it can be stated that in total $N=354$ children are diagnosed with a hereditary hearing impairment, resulting in an estimated prevalence of 30–35 per 100 000 children. This very rough estimate is based on a total number of 1.2 million children, derived from the highly uncertain target populations indicated in the questionnaire (see the Appendix) from various countries, and does not correspond to the birth cohorts 1985–1989.

Table 5.2 Prevalence of genetic hearing impairment in children born 1985–1989

Country	Sample size (N)	Hereditary hearing impairment (%)	Unknown cause (%)
Austria	32	28	22
Denmark	77	40	27
England	338	43	39
Finland	40	45	33
Ireland	43	56	21
Italy	494	22	18
Sweden	41	39	39

Table 5.2 also shows the proportion of unknown causes of hearing impairment, varying between 22–40%. It can be anticipated that the diagnostic evaluation protocol agreed upon among the representatives in the EU-CA will reduce the category of 'unknown cause', and thereby probably increase the proportion of hereditary hearing impairment (Table 5.3). Thus, it can be stated that the rough estimate of 30–35 per 100 000 children suffering from hereditary hearing impairment represents a substantial underestimate due to under-ascertainment of hereditary hearing impairment. A subdivision of non-syndromal/syndromal hereditary hearing impairment was performed, showing a higher proportion of non-syndromal hearing impairment in all the responding countries/areas.

Table 5.3 Minimal requirements for aetiological evaluation: definition of aetiological evaluation (this is an ongoing long term process as part of a surveillance programme).

1   Thorough clinical evaluation but not necessarily referral to a paediatrician
2   Thorough ENT examination, including vestibular testing at an appropriate age (test procedures proposed by Working Group III)
3   Ophthalmological referral at the time of identification — to an ophthalmologist who is aware of the associations between hearing impairment and ophthalmological signs/symptoms
4   CT scan at an appropriate age
5   Urinalysis at the time of identification and repeated after at least 10 years of age
6   ECG at least once at an appropriate age
7   Thyroid function tests (whatever available and decided by the individual physician) at an appropriate age
8   Serological testing (dependent on history) before the age of one year

Comments

This very preliminary information from the EU-CA on the epidemiology of hereditary hearing impairment, has resulted in a protocol for aetiological evaluation (Table 5.3 above). The birth cohort 1985–1989, being included in health surveillance programmes, will be subjected to this protocol as part of the surveillance of each child, and at the end of the CA it is anticipated that the prevalence of hereditary hearing impairment can be estimated appropriately. The collaboration with other representatives and groups within the EU-CA may further facilitate the identification of mutant genes causing non-syndromal or syndromal hereditary hearing impairment, which will ultimately prevent the devastating consequences of hearing impairment caused by heredity.

Appendix

1 What sort of data concerning the prevalence of permanent childhood hearing impairment do you have? (circle all the applications that are applicable to you):

   a) Data collected from clinic samples   yes   no

   b) Data collected from population study   yes   no

   c) Data collected from hearing aid users   yes   no

   d) Data collected as part of screen follow up   yes   no

   e) Data collected from school for the deaf   yes   no

   f) Data collected from school for hard of hearing yes   no

   g) Other: _____

2 Where are the children living:

   a) Geographical area:_____

   b) How big is the target population (children) in that area: _____
      thousand (approx.)

3 How do you define:

   a) Hearing impairment

_____

_____

_____

Indicate by audiometric thresholds the following categories of hearing impairment:

1 Mild _____   2 Moderate _____   3 Severe _____   4 Profound _____

   b) How do you define hearing disability?

_____

_____

_____

4 What birth cohorts do the children you have access to (question 1) represent? (circle as appropriate)

1980, 1981, 1982, 1983, 1984, 1985, 1986, 1987, 1988, 1989,

1990, 1991, 1992, 1993, 1994, 1995

Other, please specify: _____

5 Do any of your colleagues in your country have data that may be of value to this project? Please give some details about the data below:

_____

_____

_____

_____

6 Do you have any estimate for the prevalence of congenital hearing impairment (defined as permanent $\geqslant$40 dB HL in the better hearing ear, averaged across 0.5, 1, 2 and 4 kHz or equivalent) in your data for different birth cohorts, e.g. 1985–1990 or others, as defined by you?

_____

_____

_____

Is the indicated estimate:

a) A population estimate?

b) An approximate estimate based on clinical samples?

c) An informed guess?

7 Do you have any estimate for the prevalence of acquired (post-neonatally) hearing impairment (defined as permanent $\geqslant$40 dB HL in the better hearing ear, averaged across 0.5, 1, 2 and 4 kHz or equivalent) in your data for different birth cohorts, e.g. 1985–1990 or others, as defined by you?

_____

_____

_____

Is the indicated estimate:

a) A population estimate?

b) An approximate estimate based on clinical samples?

c) An informed guess?

8 For the children born with permanent hearing impairment in the birth cohort 1985–1990 (or other defined cohorts): what proportion has an aetiology of genetic origin?

        % based on $N =$ cases   or don't know

Is this:

i) Exact

ii) An approximation

iii) An informed guess

For those children with a genetic aetiology: what proportion have a hearing impairment with a syndromal manifestation?

        % based on $N =$ genetic cases   or don't know

Is this:

i) Exact

ii) An approximation

iii) An informed guess

List the diagnosed syndromes and indicate the numbers of children for each syndrome:

_____

_____

_____

What is the proportion of:

a) Dominantly inherited? _____

b) Recessively inherited? _____

c) X-linked recessive inherited? _____

d) Mitochondrially inherited? _____

Is this:

i) Exact _____

ii) An approximation _____

iii) An informed guess _____

iv) Don't know _____

Additional comments:

_____

_____

_____

_____

_____

Name and affiliation:

Chapter 6
The German Registry for Hearing Impairment in Children: preliminary results

U FINCKH-KRÄMER, ME SPORMANN-LAGODZINSKI,
A CHERECHEVSKAIA, A COSTA, E ROSZTOK, M HESS and
M GROSS

Introduction

In 1995 the German Registry for Hearing Impairment in Children started to collect medical data of children with permanent hearing impairment. The data are recorded in an ACCESS 2.0 database. Each record consists of about 100 items as numerically encoded items (e.g. sex, risk factors, type of hearing impairment), numerical values (e.g. audiometric data) or text (e.g. associated findings), if necessary.

A mailing system (to announce the number of new cases monthly), a special questionnaire and a manual (to support the users in filling in the questionnaires) have been established for all ENT, audiological or phoniatric and paedoaudiological departments and for all those specializing in diagnosis and therapy of hearing impairment. Colleagues have been asked to return answer sheets and the completed questionnaires. Trying to keep the compliance high, it was decided to condense the most important questions on to one sheet with 34 questions. For PC-equipped institutions, data may be fed directly into a PC. The software provided will create a formatted letter for patient or physician information and store the data for transfer via disk.

Method

Up to September 1996, more than 500 children had been registered throughout Germany. To obtain statistical data numerical or numerically encoded data were calculated on a weekly basis, using statistical tools developed by the staff of the Registry. The tools use classes of objects (e.g. queries, macros, reports) and functions (e.g. grouping, mean value, standard deviation) provided by ACCESS 2.0.

The following evaluation topics are presented: type of hearing impairment, hearing level, risk factors, positive family history of hearing impairment, age at first diagnosis, time lag between first suspicion and ascertained diagnosis ('diagnostic interval') time between diagnosis and beginning of therapy, probable cause of hearing impairment (hereditary/acquired/unknown), progression, therapy (e.g. hearing aid, ear surgery, cochlear implant).

The results are presented in preformatted reports as text or as figures. The underlying queries are automatically updated by ACCESS when the report is initialized. The statistical survey can be printed as hard copy or exported to other applications for further use.

Results

Up to September 1996, 26 centres had provided information about 546 children. Examples of the results are shown in Figures 6.1–6.4. About 50 new cases are registered per month. As the number of participating institutes is growing monthly, it is expected that more colleagues will become motivated to support the German Registry for Hearing Impairment in Children in order to yield the basis for future epidemiological research.

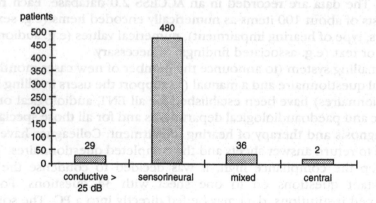

Figure 6.1 Types of hearing impairment.

Discussion

The evaluation of the first 546 records shows that persistent hearing impairment in children throughout Germany is still detected much too late (the mean age at diagnosis being more than three years). For a considerable group of children the diagnostic interval is more than one year. Further evaluation will show which groups of children have a delayed diagnosis. Our data are, in an additional cooperative project, related to epidemiological data pooled by paediatricians.

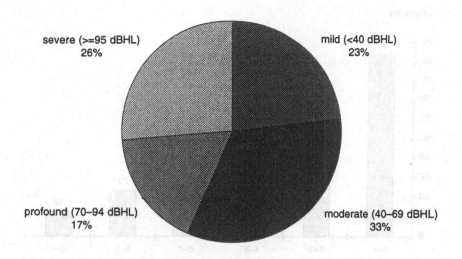

severe (>=95 dBHL)
26%

mild (<40 dBHL)
23%

profound (70–94 dBHL)
17%

moderate (40–69 dBHL)
33%

Figure 6.2 Degree of hearing impairment.

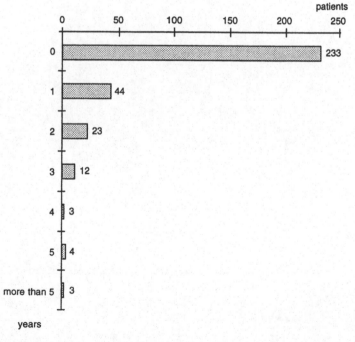

Figure 6.3 Diagnostic interval. Evaluation of all records which contain at least information about month and year of first suspicion and diagnosis of persistent hearing impairment.

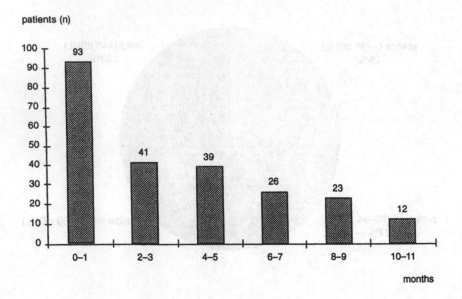

Figure 6.4 Diagnostic interval <1 year.

Chapter 7
Recessive hearing impairment in two birth cohorts in western Sicily

G GRISANTI, AM AMODEO, S CRINO and E MARTINES

Introduction

A review of epidemiological studies performed in the period 1960–1991 concerning the aetiology of childhood hearing impairment indicates that the apparent prevalence of the genetic hearing impairment has increased from 9% to 36%, with a strong increase in the last 10 years (Holten and Parving, 1985; Newton, 1985; Das 1988; Dias and Andrea, 1990; Arslan et al., 1991; Pabla et al., 1991).

The increased prevalence of genetic hearing impairment may be correlated with a parallel decrease of hearing impairment of unknown cause that has fallen from 35% to 25%.

About 50% of all profound childhood hearing impairment has a genetic aetiology although, due to diagnostic difficulties and/or to insufficient family anamnesis, this is often classified among those of unknown aetiology. About 30% of all genetic hearing impairment is part of more complex syndromes whose phenotype is characterized by different alterations in several organs (Neri and Zollino, 1992; Winter and Baraitser, 1993; Gorlin et al., 1995).

The hearing impairments with recessive inheritance represent about 60% of all genetic hearing impairments (Clementi and Tenconi, 1994). The presence of deaf siblings and normal parents, or parental consanguinity is predictive of this form of inheritance. Such a form of genetic transmission could occur directly from parents to children or indirectly across the progenitors and would be disclosed by the marriage of consanguineous subjects (David et al., 1992).

Consanguinity has a genetic significance because two parents who have a recent common ancestor may each have the same recessive gene inherited from the common ancestor. If the gene is quite rare, parental consanguinity is frequently found.

Method

This study is an epidemiological investigation of congenital recessive hearing impairment in western Sicily. Two birth cohorts of patients were examined at the Department of Audiology, University of Palermo. The first included 1293 subjects born between 1975–1979 and the second cohort included 1276 subjects born between 1985–1989. All the subjects suffered from a permanent hearing impairment defined as >40 dB HL in the better hearing ear averaged across 0.5–4 kHz.

The prevalence of the inherited hearing impairment was studied in both cohorts. In addition, among the subjects diagnosed with recessive hearing impairment the proportion of those who had consanguineous parents was calculated.

When interpreting epidemiological findings, a comparison between recessive hearing impairment/consanguinity rate in the two birth cohorts was performed.

For the diagnosis of recessive hereditary hearing impairment the following criteria were considered:

• Parental consanguinity to any degree.
• Two or more children with unaffected parents.
• Only child with unaffected parents but with affected cousin(s).
• Pedigree suggesting recessive inheritance.

Results

No significant differences in the prevalence of inherited hearing impairment were found between the two cohorts 1975–1979 and 1985–1989, accounting for 0.067% (136 cases/201 971 target population) and 0.058% (111 cases/189 500 target population), respectively (Figure 7.1).

Furthermore, among the number of inherited hearing impairments in the samples, the percentage of recessive hearing impairment was calculated. This was similar in the two cohorts accounting for 84.6% (Figure 7.2) and 81.1% (Figure 7.3), respectively.

Significant differences were found between the two birth cohorts 1975–1979 and 1985–1989 in the recessive hearing impairment/consanguinity rate.

The percentage of the subjects with recessive hearing impairment and parental consanguinity was 41.7% and 21.1% (Figure 7.4) in the two birth cohorts, respectively.

It is noteworthy that a 50% decrease does not correspond to a decrease in recessive hearing impairment. Thus it would seem that genetic counselling may be a useful tool to reduce the prevalence of recessive hearing impairment, and should be supported by alternative strategies to reduce this kind of hearing impairment.

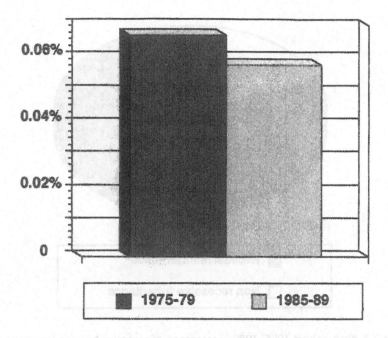

Figure 7.1 Birth cohorts 1975–1979 and 1985–1989: prevalence of inherited hearing impairment.

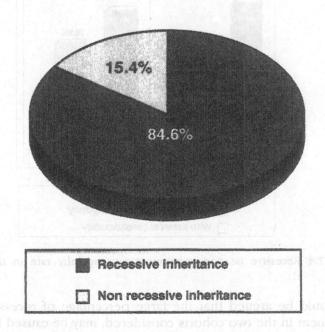

Figure 7.2 Birth cohort 1975–1979: percentage of recessive hearing impairment.

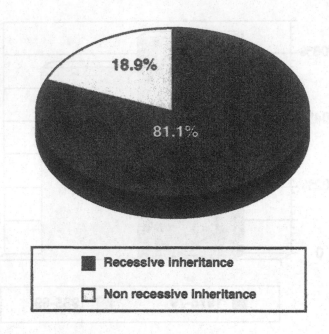

Figure 7.3 Birth cohort 1985–1989: percentage of recessive hearing impairment.

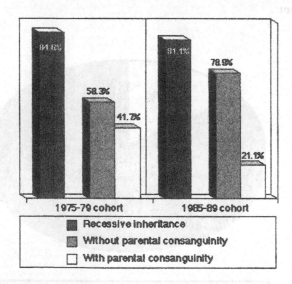

Figure 7.4 Recessive hearing impairment/consanguinity rate in the two birth cohorts.

It could be argued that the large percentage of recessive hearing impairment in the two cohorts considered, may be caused by the large number of carriers in the population of western Sicily in which, until recently, consanguineous marriages were quite common.

Conclusions

Two birth cohorts of patients were examined at the Department of Audiology, University of Palermo. The first included 1293 subjects born between 1975–1979 and the second cohort included 1276 subjects born between 1985–1989. All the subjects suffered from a permanent hearing impairment defined as >40 dB HL in the better hearing ear.

In both cohorts, inheritance was the most common cause of congenital hearing impairment and transmission was recessive.

A comparison between recessive hearing impairment/consanguinity rate in the two birth cohorts indicated significant differences.

Acknowledgement

This study was supported by grants from the Italian Ministero dell'Università e della Ricerca Scientifica e Tecnologica.

Chapter 8
Aetiology of hearing impairment in children born in northern Finland in 1975–1979 and in 1985–1989.

E MÄKI-TORKKO, P LINDHOLM, M VÄYRYNEN and M SORRI

Abstract

The aetiology of hearing impairment, and the genetic causes, in particular, were studied in a clinical series in northern Finland. All children with permanent hearing impairment on pure tone average (PTA) 0.5–4 kHz $\geq$ 50 dB HL in the better hearing ear who had been born between 1975–1979 (Group I, 50 children) and 1985–1989 (Group II, 39 children) and belonged to the Oulu University Hospital service area were included in the series. Children with infectious aetiology were excluded. All children with this degree of hearing impairment in this population are diagnosed and have their rehabilitation started in the Oulu University Hospital. The patient records of each child were reviewed retrospectively.

The mean better ear hearing level was 86.7 dB HL (SD 23.8 dB HL) for the older age group and 82.3 dB HL (SD 21.0 dB HL) for the younger, and the prevalences were 0.9/1000 and 0.8/1000, respectively. The median age at diagnosis was 2.3 years in the older group and 2.0 years in the younger, indicating only a slight improvement over 10 years. Group I included eight children with non-syndromal and six children with syndromal familial hearing impairment, and the corresponding figures in Group II were 12 and six, respectively. With regard to both non-syndromal and syndromal hearing impairments, five dominant, seven recessive and one unknown form of inheritance and one chromosomal abnormality were found in Group I. In addition to three cases of dominant, eight of recessive and five of unknown forms of inheritance, there was one case with X-linked inheritance in Group II.

Although the number of subjects is small, the most common genetic syndrome was found to be the Usher syndrome, with two cases in

Group I and three in Group II. The other causes included adverse peri-
natal factors, meningitis, non-genetic syndromes, ear anomalies and
rubella. It is worth pointing out that the rubella vaccination programme,
established in 1975 in Finland, has been successful and the number of
children with a hearing impairment caused by maternal rubella infection had decreased from six to one in the series. The aetiology was
unknown for 19 (38.0%) subjects in the older group and 13 (33.3%) in
the younger. In view of the unknown aetiologies, further research is
warranted and the possibility of maternally inherited mitochondrial
defects has also to be taken into consideration. The proportion of inherited hearing impairments had increased from 28% in those born
between 1975–1979 to 44% in those born between 1985–1989. This is
likely to be due to the improved diagnostic methods, since we found
some decrease in the amount of unknown causes within the same
period. Nowadays parents also seem to be more willing to find out the
cause of their child's impairment and to attend genetic consultation
more often than they did some years ago.

PART V
AUDIOVESTIBULAR TESTS

Chapter 9
Audiometric criteria for linkage analysis in genetic hearing impairment

FL WUYTS, PH VAN DE HEYNING and F DECLAU

Introduction

For a successful linkage analysis, a careful selection of genetically affected and non-affected members is essential. The basic condition for conducting a successful search for genetic loci responsible for sensorineural hearing impairment, is the identification of individuals with a similar phenotype. This is based on careful history, and clinical examination and after the exclusion of suspected or identifiable non-hereditary causes on their audiometric threshold profile. We here propose an audiological method for including and excluding individuals in a linkage analysis study. This method proved to be successful in the mapping of DFNA2 (Coucke et al., 1994, Van Camp et al., 1997) in several families.

Method

Initially, hearing impairment from non-genetic causes of hearing impairment or from environmental factors, such as excessive noise exposure, ototoxic drugs, infection as well as injury were excluded by the different diagnostic techniques including audiometry. The age of onset was studied by pedigree analysis. The upper limit was denoted as the cut-off age.

To differentiate between genetically affected and non-affected members in a given family, the p95 and p50 threshold levels of an otologically normal population were used. The p95 value, representing the auditory threshold exceeded by only 5% of a normal population, was chosen to limit the error of including a member with an apparently 'affected' audiological profile but generated by variability of nature. The p95 limit was calculated for each frequency tested and the p50 adopted from the ISO7029 (ISO, 1984) criteria, which offer guidelines for calculating the percentile hearing threshold values for an otologically normal population. In this international standard, otologically normal individuals comprised people in a normal state of health who, at the time of testing, were free from excess wax in the ear canal, and without known ear pathology nor history of undue exposure to noise. The hearing threshold is determined by means of a pure tone air conduction audiometer, expressed as the hearing level in decibels.

Different calculation coefficients exist for gender, age and frequency. To calculate the p95 values, the following formula was derived from the ISO7029 guidelines:

$$H(p95,y) = 1.732*a*(y-18)^n2 + 1.645*bu$$

In this equation, y represents the age in years of the subject and a(dB/year) and bu (dB) are constants depending on gender and tone frequency (Table 9.1).

Table 9.1 Constants a(dB/year) and bu by gender and frequency (ISO7029)

Frequency (Hz)	a Males	a Females	bu Males	bu Females
125	0.003	0.003	7.23	6.67
250	0.003	0.003	6.67	6.12
500	0.0035	0.0035	6.12	6.12
1000	0.004	0.004	6.12	6.12
1500	0.0055	0.005	6.67	6.67
2000	0.007	0.006	7.23	6.67
3000	0.0115	0.0075	7.78	7.23
4000	0.016	0.009	8.34	7.78
6000	0.018	0.012	9.45	8.9
8000	0.022	0.015	10.56	10.56

The pedigree member was assumed to be genetically affected if the hearing threshold of at least two frequencies for both ears exceeded the p95 limit. This rule was applied to take into account the measurement error of the audiometric threshold determination. The pedigree member was included in the non-affected group, if the audiometric threshold profile was better than the p50 value for all frequencies, and if the subject was older than the cut-off age.

Results

Tables 9.2 and 9.3 show the p95 values for male and female subjects for the ages 20–70 years, for the frequencies 125–8000 Hz. Tables 9.4 and 9.5 show the p50 values as reported in the ISO7029 guidelines.

Table 9.2 p95 audiological threshold levels (dBA) for normal male subjects

Male age (years)				Frequency (Hz)				
	125	250	500	1000	2000	3000	4000	6000	8000
20	12	11	10	10	12	13	14	16	18
30	13	12	11	11	14	16	18	20	23
40	14	13	13	13	18	22	27	31	36
50	17	16	16	17	24	33	42	47	56
60	21	20	21	22	33	48	63	71	85
70	26	25	26	29	·45	67	89	100	120

Table 9.3 p95 audiological threshold levels (dBA) for normal female subjects

Female age (years)				Frequency (Hz)				
	125	250	500	1000	2000	3000	4000	6000	8000
20	11	10	10	10	11	12	13	15	17
30	12	11	11	11	12	14	15	18	21
40	13	13	13	13	16	18	20	25	30
50	16	15	16	17	22	25	29	36	44
60	20	19	21	22	29	35	40	51	63
70	25	24	26	29	39	47	55	71	88

Table 9.4 p50 audiological threshold levels (dBA) for normal male subjects

Male age (years)				Frequency (Hz)				
	125	250	500	1000	2000	3000	4000	6000	8000
20	0	0	0	0	0	0	0	0	0
30	0	0	1	1	1	2	2	3	3
40	1	1	2	2	3	6	8	9	11
50	3	3	4	4	7	12	16	18	23
60	5	5	6	7	12	20	28	32	39
70	8	8	9	11	19	31	43	49	60

Table 9.5 p50 audiological threshold levels (dBA) for normal female subjects

Female age (years)				Frequency (Hz)				
	125	250	500	1000	2000	3000	4000	6000	8000
20	0	0	0	0	0	0	0	0	0
30	0	0	1	1	1	1	1	2	2
40	1	1	2	2	3	4	4	6	7
50	3	3	4	4	6	8	9	12	15
60	5	5	6	7	11	13	16	21	27
70	8	8	9	11	16	20	24	32	41

Figures 9.1–9.4 are the audiometric representations of the p50 and p95 values for both sexes, for each decade.

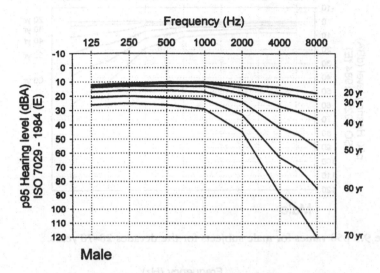

Figure 9.1 p95 values for male subjects for the decades 20–70 years.

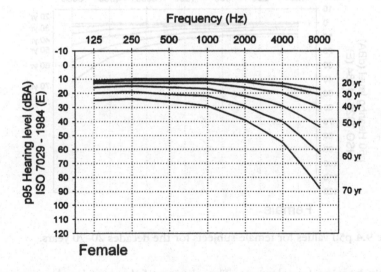

Figure 9.2 p95 values for female subjects for the decades 20–70 years.

Discussion

An audiometric strategy is proposed to differentiate between genetically affected and non-affected members in families with a progressive non-syndromal sensorineural hearing impairment.

Based upon the p95 and p50 values, criteria for inclusion and exclusion are provided for linkage analysis in families suspected of having

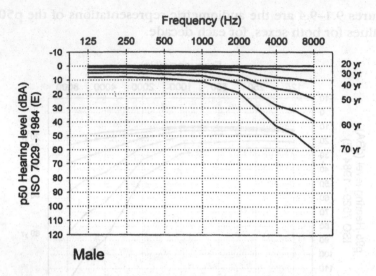

Figure 9.3 p50 values for male subjects for the decades 20–70 years.

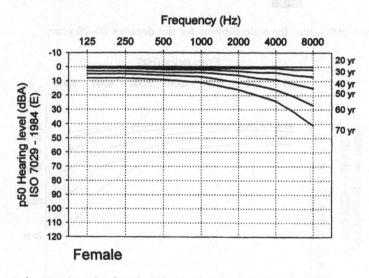

Figure 9.4 p50 values for female subjects for the decades 20–70 years.

genetic hearing impairment. The choice of the two levels, worse than p95 for the affected and better than p50 for the non-affected members, yields a high specificity and sensitivity. The disadvantage of the method consists of a relatively large number of individuals who cannot be classified and hence are not included in the linkage analysis. However, this disadvantage is balanced out by the deleterious effect on the lod-score of misclassification. This methodology has proved to be successful for the gene mapping of DFNA2 (Coucke et al., 1994; Van Camp et al., 1997) in several families.

Conclusions

The audiological strategy for the successful mapping of the deafness gene DFNA2 in several families is reported. Proper inclusion and exclusion criteria of pedigree members is paramount for mapping non-syndromal sensorineural hearing impairment. These inclusion criteria are based upon comparison of their hearing threshold levels with normative thresholds for subjects of the same age and gender with exclusion of other suspected or identified causes. Hearing worse than the p95 limit has been chosen for the inclusion of subjects as being phenotypically hearing impaired. Hearing less than the p50 limit was adopted for the inclusion in the linkage analysis of the non-affected subjects, on condition that they are older than the maximum onset or cut-off age of the disease. Based on the ISO7029 (ISO, 1984) guidelines for age- and gender-related hearing impairment, the p95 has been calculated in detail for males and females, for the decades between 20–70 years.

Chapter 10
Audioscan notches in carriers of genetic hearing impairment

F ZHAO, D STEPHENS, R MEREDITH and VE NEWTON

Introduction

The audioscan is a form of high definition audiometry based on constant hearing level frequency sweeps. It can detect slight audiometric disorders, such as narrow notches, situated between the frequencies normally tested (Meyer Bisch, 1996). Such notches have been shown to be more common in the carriers of certain genetic hearing impairments (Meredith, 1991; Stephens et al., 1995; Stephens and Francis, 1996), and also in normally hearing people with tinnitus (Sirimanna et al., 1996). However, the reliability of this technique has been called into question. Some authors have obtained less consistent results by the use of different stimulus parameters and criteria for notches (Cohen et al., 1996a; Wagenaar et al., 1996). These have included the use of different sweep rates. Therefore, a precise protocol and fixed criterion for the notches are crucial for comparing the findings of different studies.

A pilot study by Meredith (1991) indicated that audioscan notches were found less frequently in a group of three subjects when tested with fast sweep rates (10 and 20 s/octave) than at slower sweep rates (30 and 40 s/octave).

In the present study, the influence of sweep rate on the reliability of notches found on audioscan testing was investigated in order to establish standard stimulus parameters for the detection of subclinical cochlear pathology (Study 1). The characteristics of notches found in 100 subjects were also investigated in order to define better criteria for notches and the parameters for describing them (Study 2).

Method

Subjects

Study 1

Twelve subjects, selected from among members of staff and students in Cardiff and Manchester, were studied to test the influence of sweep rate on the reliability of notches. All had been found to have normal hearing, but notches on audioscan testing. Two sweep rates, 15 versus 30 s/octave were used in the study. The subjects were tested on two occasions as follows:

* First visit: starting with 15 s/octave, followed by 30 s/octave.
* Second visit: starting with 30 s/octave, followed by 15 s/octave.

In alternate subjects (i.e. odd/even numbers) the order was reversed.

Study 2

* Normal control subjects: 11 normal control subjects found to have notches were drawn from hospital staff, visitors and medical students.
* Carriers of Usher II syndrome: 12 parents or siblings of three patients with Usher II syndrome who had been found to have notches on audioscan testing.
* Carriers of non-syndromal autosomal recessive hearing impairment: 77 parents or siblings in 58 families where one or more of the children had a non-acquired hearing impairment who had been found to have notches on audioscan testing.

Audioscan

The audioscan test was carried out using the Essilor Audioscan. The test parameters were as follows:

* Frequency range: 300–4000 Hz.
* Starting level: −5 dB.
* Sweep rate: 30 s/octave or 15 s/octave[1].
* Start side: right.
* Stimulus style: pulsed tone.
* Step size: 5 dB.

Notch measurement

The parameters of notch measurement (Figure 10.1) were recommended by Laroche and Hétu (1997) as follows:
* Centre frequency (F): corresponds to the frequency of the deepest point of the notch.

---

[1] 15 s/octave was only used in Study 1.

- Starting point (*S*): the best hearing threshold preceding the notch.
- Absolute value in dB (*N*): represents the absolute value of the notch lower extremity expressed in dB measured at *F*.
- Depth (*P*): the difference between *N* and *S*.
- Width at 50% of depth (*W*): is determined using 50% of the total notch depth; it is measured as a proportion of an octave.

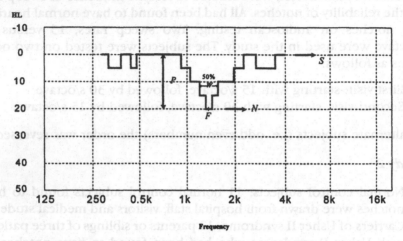

Figure 10.1 The parameters of notches.

Working definition of audioscan notch

By use of the audioscan technique, a significant notch was defined as being 15 dB or more deeper than the surrounding frequencies with the notch width not entering into the criterion (Meredith, 1991).

Results and discussion

Study 1

On experimental testing at 30 s/octave, 27/28 (96%) possible notches were found. Only on one retest was a notch not present. Testing at 15 s/octave showed only 10/28 (36%) notches (Figure 10.2). Five of 12 subjects showed no significant notches on either test at this sweep rate. A χ^2 test showed that the reliability of notches at 30 s/octave was significantly better than at 15 s/octave ($\chi^2 = 23.0$; d.f. = 1; $p < 0.0005$). This indicates that the reliability with the slower sweep speed was better than that with fast speed and is in keeping with the findings in the pilot study by Meredith (1991), who showed that 100% notches were present at 30 and 40 s/octave, but that only 25% were present at 10 and 20 s/octave in three subjects with notches in both ears.

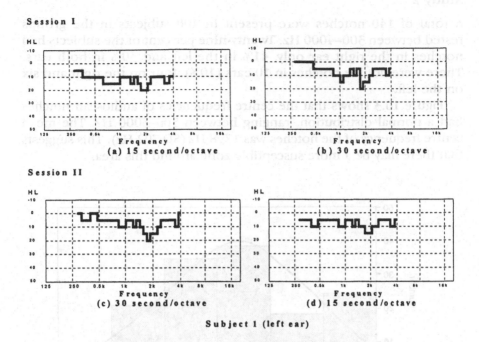

Session I

(a) 15 second/octave

(b) 30 second/octave

Session II

(c) 30 second/octave

(d) 15 second/octave

Subject 1 (left ear)

Figure 10.2 Example of audioscan tests on the two occasions.

In addition, the parameters of the notches were assessed at the different sweep rates on the two occasions. Table 10.1 shows the means of the main parameters of the notches. At the sweep rate of 30 s/octave the notch centre frequencies obtained in the two tests were significantly correlated between tests ($rho = 0.93$; $p < 0.0005$). Moreover, notch centre frequencies at 30 s/octave also correlated significantly with those of the notches found at 15 s/octave ($rho = 0.97$; $p < 0.0005$). No such significant correlations were found in the width and depth of the notches ($p > 0.05$) either between two occasions tested at 30 s/octave or between two different sweep rates.

Table 10.1 Means ± SD of the main parameters of audioscan notches tested at 30 s/octave and 15 s/octave on the two occasions

	Centre frequency (Hz)	Depth (dB)	Width (1/9 octave)
At 30 s/octave			
1st visit	2142 ± 476	15.4 ± 1.4	4.1 ± 2.7
2nd visit	2119 ± 468	16.4 ± 2.3	4.5 ± 2.0
At 15 s/octave			
1st visit	1959 ± 482	15.0 ± 0.0	3.7 ± 2.7
2nd visit	2210 ± 336	16.3 ± 2.5	3.2 ± 1.5

Study 2

A total of 140 notches were present in 100 subjects in the groups tested between 300–4000 Hz. Twenty-nine per cent of the subjects had notches in the right ear only, 41% in the left and 30% in both ears. There were double notches in 10 ears (10%), four on the right and six on the left.

Figure 10.3 shows that the centre frequencies of audioscan notches had a normal distribution, ranging between 500–3000 Hz. The mean centre frequency of the notches was 1798 Hz (SD 702 Hz). This suggests that there may be a more susceptible zone around this area.

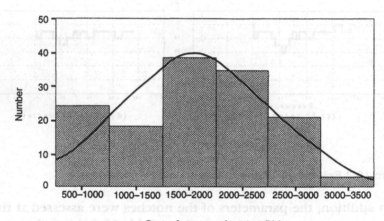

Centre frequency of notches (Hz)

Figure 10.3 Distribution of centre frequencies of audioscan notches.

The width of the notches of the subjects tested over the frequency range 300–4000 Hz was log-normally distributed. The geometric mean, median and modal width was 1/3 octave (Figure 10.4).

Figure 10.5 shows the distribution of the depths of audioscan notches, 71.4 % of the notches were 15 dB deep, 24.3% 20 dB deep and only 4.3% 25 dB or more deep.

Furthermore, over three-quarters of notches started between –5 and +5 dB HL (Figure 10.6). In 22 subjects (total 31 notches) this starting point was at –5 dB. Of those in whom the starting level was at –5 dB HL, 74.2% had a depth of 15 dB, 16.1 of 20 dB and 9.7% 25 dB or more. This implies that starting testing at 0 dB HL would result in 16.4% of all notches being missed.

Table 10.2 shows that, in the 30 subjects with bilateral notches, there was a significant correlation (Spearman *rho*) between the notch depths of the two ears (*rho* = 0.42; *p*<0.05), but not between the centre frequencies and widths.

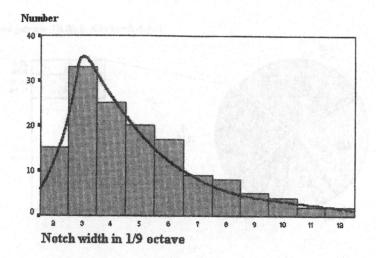

Figure 10.4 Width distribution of notches.

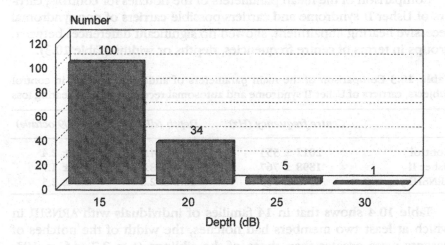

Figure 10.5 Distribution of depths of audioscan notches.

Table 10.2 Main parameters of audioscan notches in subjects with bilateral notches and the correlations between the ears

	Centre frequency (Hz)	*Depth (dB)*	*Width (1/9 octave)*
Right ear	1767 ± 784	16.5 ± 2.7	4.9 ± 5.6
Left ear	1734 ± 615	16.8 ± 3.6	4.3 ± 2.7
rho	0.15	0.42	−0.08
p	NS	0.05	NS

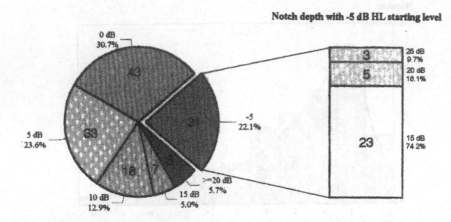

Figure 10.6 Starting levels of the notches.

Comparison of the mean parameters of the notches for controls, carriers of Usher II syndrome and carriers/possible carriers of non-syndromal recessive hearing impairment, showed no significant differences between groups in terms of centre frequencies, depths or widths (Table 10.3).

Table 10.3 Comparison of the main parameters of audioscan notches in control subjects, carriers of Usher II syndrome and autosomal recessive genetic hearing loss

	Centre frequency (Hz)	*Depth (dB)*	*Width (1/9 octave)*
Control	2012 ± 553	16.6 ± 4.7	4.1 ± 2.4
Usher II	1898 ± 767	17.9 ± 8.7	3.4 ± 1.7
ARNSHI	1748 ± 709	16.6 ± 2.8	4.0 ± 2.5

Table 10.4 shows that in 14 families of individuals with ARNSHI in which at least two members had notches, the width of the notches of parents were greater than those of the siblings ($t = 2.7$, d.f. $= 103$; $p<0.01$). There were no significant differences in the centre frequencies or depths. Analysis of variance showed no significant differences within or between family effects for any of the other parameters.

Table 10.4 Comparison of the main parameters of audioscan notches between parents and siblings

	Centre frequency (Hz)	*Depth (dB)*	*Width (1/9 octave)*
Parents	1807 ± 719	16.4 ± 2.4	4.5 ± 2.6
Siblings	1647 ± 687	16.8 ± 3.3	3.2 ± 2.0*

*$p<0.01$

Conclusions

The reliability of notches detected with a sweep rate of 30 seconds per octave was significantly better than that at 15 s/octave.

Five of 12 subjects failed to show notches at all when tested at 15 s/octave although all had notches when tested at 30 s/octave.

A precise experimental protocol and notch definition are crucial for comparing the findings of different studies with audioscan.

Well-defined parameters of notches allow us to investigate the reproducibility of audioscan tests and to compare the characteristics of the notches in different clinical contexts.

There were no significant differences in the main parameters of notches found between control subjects, carriers of Usher II syndrome and possible carriers of non-syndromal autosomal recessive hearing impairment.

If the starting level is set at 0 dB HL rather than –5 dB HL, 16.4% of all notches would be missed.

Chapter 11
Cochlear irregularities in obligate carriers of recessive genetic hearing impairment and in control subjects

G LINA-GRANADE, M KREISS, T GELAS, L COLLET and
A MORGON

Introduction

Genetic hearing impairment (GHI) is probably the most important cause of childhood sensorineural hearing impairment. Among genetic hearing impairment, the autosomal recessive mode of inheritance is the most frequent as well as that most usually responsible for profound congenital hearing impairment (Reardon, 1992).

These recessive hearing impairments are difficult to diagnose when there is only one affected child in a family. Therefore, about one-third of all profound prelingual hearing impairments remains with no known aetiology. The consequence is that no accurate genetic counselling can be given to the parents.

In order that these cases can be labelled, a means of determining whether the parents are carriers of autosomal recessive hearing impairment (ARHI) (or if the mother is carrier of X-linked deafness, although this is much rarer) is needed.

Several studies have reported mild auditory anomalies in obligate carriers of ARHI. Audiometric notches have been detected in all tested obligate carriers of Usher syndrome and Alport syndrome, and in about 66% of obligate carriers of non-syndromal autosomal recessive hearing impairment (NSARHI) (Meredith et al., 1992; Sirimanna et al., 1994; Stephens et al., 1995).

Transient-evoked otoacoustic emissions (TEOAEs), which are thought to reflect outer hair cell activity (Probst et al., 1991), were found to be significantly lower for the 500–1500 Hz spectrum band, in a group of obligate carriers of ARHI compared to a group of control subjects (Cohen et al., 1996b).

The present study was designed to:

- Determine the prevalence of such audiometric notches in French obligate carriers of autosomal recessive hearing impairment (ARHI).
- Compare it to a control subject population.
- Establish if these notches reflect cochlear irregularities by studying their test–retest reproducibility, and by comparing them with transient-evoked otoacoustic emissions.

Method

Obligate carriers

Fifteen subjects were included in this group: nine women and six men (21–44 years old), from nine families. Criteria for obligate carriers were:

- Parents of more than two hearing impaired children (10 subjects).
- Child of a hearing impaired parent who had affected siblings and normally hearing parents (one subject).
- Parents with one affected child and two affected relatives with severe or profound prelingual hearing impairment (four subjects).

Hearing impairment in affected relatives had no obvious extrinsic cause. Only 14 carriers underwent audiometry, all had TEOAE recordings.

Control subjects

This group included 50 normally hearing subjects with no family history of hearing impairment, no noise exposure and no otological history. Twenty-two subjects were men, 28 were women; their ages ranged between 18–49 years (mean 25.6 years). Only forty control subjects performed high definition audiometry; all 50 subjects underwent TEOAE recordings.

Procedures

High-definition audiometry was performed with an audioscan (Essilor) audiometer, in a sound-attenuating chamber. Subjective thresholds to 64 frequencies per octave, between 300–4000 Hz, were obtained. The sweep rate was 30 s/octave. The test always began with the right ear at 0 dB HL.

Audiometric notches were defined as a frequency region where threshold is more than 15 dB below thresholds at neighbouring frequencies (Figure 11.1).

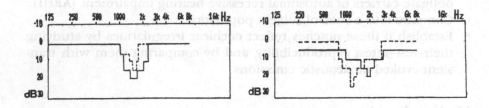

Figure 11.1 Examples of reproducible high-definition audiometry notches. Solid and dashed lines represent the result of two tests for a given ear.

TEOAE recordings were performed with an ILO88 probe, software and hardware (Otodynamics, London), in a sound-attenuating chamber.

The responses to 500 unfiltered clicks at 80 dB pe SPL were averaged. The TEOAE spectrum was studied in 49-Hz bands between extreme frequencies with detectable TEOAEs (0.5–4.5 kHz maximum).

TEOAE notches were defined as a group of successive frequency bands where TEOAE amplitude was <3 dB above the noise, or >10 dB below the amplitude at the neighbouring frequencies (three frequency bands below and three above the considered frequency) (Figure 11.2). Notches were automatically detected by transfer of TEOAE data to a purpose-made program on Microsoft ExcelR.

Reproducibility: in control subjects, high-definition audiometry and otoacoustic emission recordings were repeated twice to assess test–retest reproducibility. The tests were conducted with repositioning of headphones or probe, within an interval of 30 min to several days. The stimulus level for TEOAE recording was identical ±0.8 dB on all recordings for a given ear.

An audiometric notch was considered as reproducible if it included at least some common frequencies (see Figure 11.1 above). TEOAE reproducible notches were defined as notches present on both recordings of one ear at the same frequency ±49 Hz.

Results

Audiometric notches

Nineteen control subjects of the 40 (48%) had an audiometric notch (it was unilateral in all but two subjects). Notch width ranged between less than half an octave to two octaves. The proportion of reproducible notches among the total number of notches for the 40 subjects was 40%. So only 16% of control subjects had a reproducible notch. Gender did

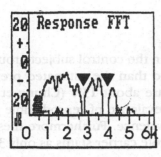 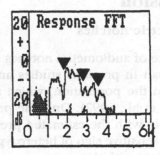

Figure 11.2 Examples of notches in the TEOAE spectrum (indicated by arrows). Horizontal axis: frequency (kHz); vertical axis: amplitude (dB). Left: notches where TEOAE amplitude is <3 dB above noise; Right: notches where TEOAE amplitude is >10 dB below amplitude at the neighbouring frequencies (three frequency bands below or three frequency bands above the frequency considered).

not influence the presence of notches. Among the 14 obligate carriers of ARHI, five (36%) had an audiometric notch.

Notches in TEOAE spectrum

All ears in both groups had notches in the TEOAE spectrum as defined by mathematical criteria. Most (65%) of these notches were only 49 Hz wide. In control subjects, 80% of these notches were reproducible.

The total number of TEOAE notches did not differ significantly between carriers and age-matched control subjects, except for the number of notches in the 500–1500 Hz range ($p=0.0001$). Yet, most obligate carriers (9/15) had a number of notches in the 500–1500 Hz range which were included in the confidence interval defined in controls (mean ±2 SD). TEOAE total amplitude was not significantly different between the two groups.

Correlation between TEOAEs and reproducible audiometric notches

In control subjects, only six audiometric notches were related to EOAE notches at the same frequency (same frequency for the lowest EOAE amplitude and the worst audiometric threshold) and two were related to within 300 Hz.

In carriers, two audiometric notches out of five were related to EOAE notches at the same frequency.

Most TEOAE notches, even if wide, were not related to an audiometric notch or to poorer audiometric thresholds.

Discussion

Audiometric notches

Prevalence of audiometric notches in the control subject group is much higher than in previous studies and than the estimated prevalence of carriers in the population, which are about 13% (Chung et al., 1959; Meredith et al., 1992). Only the prevalence of reproducible notches is compatible with the estimated prevalence. Furthermore these notches are not a sensitive sign of heterozygote carrier status as only 36% of carriers present with them.

These differences, as compared with previous studies, might stem from the different ethnic and genetic background of the subjects tested, and from different genes of ARHI in the various carriers (various degrees of hearing impairment in affected relatives).

A technical origin might also be implied: the low reproducibility of audiometric notches can be explained by the high dependence of audiometry on test conditions (background noise, instructions, subject attention and training). Two arguments support this explanation: most non-reproducible notches were correlated with a less deep notch on the other test, and most non-reproducible notches were on the first test of the right ear (75%), i.e. on the first recording.

Reproducibility might probably be better if the subjects were trained to hear the test tones before starting the test, if background noise was completely avoided, and if the test was interrupted at the first sign of declining attention.

The need for two successive tests when a 10 or 15 dB notch is detected has also to be considered.

Notches in TEOAE spectrum

TEOAE notches have a high reproducibility, suggesting that they reflect physiological irregularities.

The only statistical difference between carriers and controls (number of notches in the 500–1500 Hz range) is in the same frequency range as the amplitude difference found in a previous study (Cohen et al., 1996b). However, that statistical difference does not permit the detection of carriers, as most of them were in the confidence interval established in control subjects.

The absence of a significant correlation between audiometric and TEOAE notches is easy to understand, as several studies have shown that correlation between subjective thresholds and TEOAE amplitude for each frequency band is not strict, and that TEOAE amplitude for each frequency band is influenced by the whole audiogram (Collet et al.,

1992). Moreover, the presence of notches might be influenced by spontaneous otoacoustic emissions, which were not tested, and which are not correlated with audiometric thresholds. Finally, the presence of TEOAEs at frequencies at which subjective thresholds are altered might reflect an isolated inner hair cell loss with normal outer hair cells (Bonfils et al., 1991).

Conclusions

Auditory irregularities found in carriers seem to be neither sensitive nor specific. Stricter experimental conditions for high-definition audiometry have to be used to improve specificity.

TEOAEs have the advantage of providing an objective test. Further TEOAE assessment might provide the opportunity of detecting carriers of ARHI. In particular, TEOAE notch width should be studied.

A combination of both tests might be the optimal way of detecting carriers of ARHI, including perhaps other auditory tests such as distortion-product otoacoustic emissions, psychoacoustical tests or extended high frequency audiometry.

Finally, genotyping of tested subjects might explain the incomplete prevalence of audiometric notches and help us to understand the physiological basis of these notches.

Chapter 12
Three-dimensional video-oculography for the detection of genetic vestibular dysfunction at the level of the three semicircular canals and the otoliths

FL WUYTS, PH VAN DE HEYNING, H KINGMA, L BOUMANS and D VAN DYCK

Abstract

Using a newly developed second generation three-dimensional video-oculographic system (3D VOG), the investigation of all the components of the vestibular system becomes possible. For the investigation of patients with genetic deficits, the refined technique of 3D VOG may elicit partial vestibular dysfunction according to the site within the vestibular organ, and or differentiate between types of genetic hearing loss based on the concomitant vestibular lesion.

The vestibular system plays a key role in the control of posture and balance, as well as in gaze stabilization during head movements. The vestibulo-ocular reflex (VOR), arising from vestibular stimulation, triggers the eye movements in order to counteract the head movement resulting in gaze stabilization. Vestibular dysfunction leads to vertigo, lateropulsion and oscillopsia.

The vestibular system consists of three semicircular canals (SCC) for the measurement of head rotation and of the utricle and saccule for linear acceleration as well as gravity detection through the otoliths. The utricle is orientated in approximately the same plane as the horizontal semicircular canals and senses antero-posterior and latero-lateral translations as well as tilts of the head. The saccule is oriented vertically and detects antero-posterior and cranio-caudal translations of the head as well as head tilts. During cranio-caudal translations the saccule is excited more than the utricle. With sustained head tilt, the eyes counter-roll, presumably as part of an attempt to align the horizontal meridian of the retina with the horizon. This reflex is mostly vestigial in human beings, the gain being only 0.1–0.2 (Zee and Hain, 1993).

Up to now, the study of the VOR in the clinical environment has been confined to the horizontal VOR by use of an electronystagmographic (ENG) recording technique following different vestibular stimuli. The contribution of the vertical and posterior SCC as well as the utricle and saccule to the VOR cannot be recorded by standard ENG. As only one-fifth of the vestibular system is tested, the high number (30–40%) of normal ENG results in patients with vertigo is to be expected.

Using a newly developed second generation 3D VOG the investigation and quantification of all the components of the VOR becomes possible. 3D VOG is based on the real-time image analysis at 50 Hz of the video-recorded eye and decomposes the eye movements into horizontal, vertical and rotational components. The second generation device is an upgraded version of the system described by Kingma et al. (1995), Kingma (1997) and Kingma et al. (1997). Apart from the updating of the frame grabbers, the eye–camera distance has been largely increased in order to improve the depth of field, sharpness and accuracy in non-central gaze. New software has eliminated the effect of pseudo-rotation.

The function of the statolith system can be evaluated by means of the static component of the eye torsion induced by body roll, eccentric rotation or latero-lateral translation. The function of the vertical and posterior semi-circular canals is tested in dynamic rotations in the sagittal pitch and frontal roll plane.

Instruction or alertness of the subject do not seem to affect the static reflex, thus allowing objective measurement of the statolith function (Van Rijn, 1994).

For the investigation of patients with genetic deficits, the refined technique of 3D VOG may elicit partial vestibular dysfunction according to the site within the vestibular organ, and/or differentiate between types of genetic hearing impairment based on the concomitant vestibular lesion. It is known that hereditary and congenital disorders can occur with or without vestibular dysfunction. With cochleo-saccular (Scheibe) dysplasia the cochlea and the saccule are involved, but not the utricle nor the semicircular canals. In Waardenburg syndrome vestibular hypofunction is frequently detected. (Rosenhall, 1996). So far, only classical vestibular testing has been used for the assessment of these vestibular dysfunctions. By use of the more precise technique of

3D VOG, the function of the vestibular sub-systems can be examined, leading to a better knowledge and/or detection of the hereditary disorders.

Acknowledgement

This work was supported by NFWO grant no. 3.0305.96.

PART VI
NON-SYNDROMAL AUTOSOMAL RECESSIVE HEARING IMPAIRMENT

Chapter 13
Homozygosity mapping applied to hereditary hearing impairment — localizing recessive deafness genes

RJH SMITH, A RAMESH, CR SRIKUMARI SRISAILAPATHY,
K FUKUSHIMA, S WAYNE, A CHEN, L VAN LAER, J ASHLEY,
RIS ZBAR, M LOVETT and G VAN CAMP

Introduction

Hearing impairment is a symptom of inner ear dysfunction. Its aetiology is multifactorial, and it affects people without regard to age, race or socio-economic background. In the USA, approximately 1/1000 neonates is born with hearing impairment sufficient in magnitude to preclude normal speech development (Fraser, 1976), and by puberty, an equal number of adolescents are similarly affected (Morton, 1991). With advancing years, median hearing thresholds decline insidiously to the extent that nearly one-half of octogenarians experience significant hearing loss (Roberts, 1968).

Several classification schemes can be applied to hearing impairment. By audiometric criteria, losses can be diagnosed as conductive, sensorineural or mixed, and graded as mild (26–40 dB), moderate (41–55 dB), moderately severe (56–70 dB), severe (71–90 dB) or profound (>90 dB) (Goodman, 1965). By anamnesis, impairments can be classified as prelingual (congenital) or post-lingual (late-in-onset), and inherited or acquired. Inherited impairments can be subclassified as syndromal or non-syndromal to reflect the presence or absence of coinherited physical abnormalities (Smith, 1986).

Among hearing impaired children, surveys suggest that the aetiology of profound hearing impairment is equally divided between inherited and acquired causes, with nearly 70% of inherited cases being autosomal recessive and non-syndromal (autosomal recessive non-syndromal hearing impairment ARNSHI) (Chung et al., 1959; Fraser, 1965: Chung and Brown, 1970; Nance et al., 1977). Segregation analysis of non-consanguineous and consanguineous marriages implicates monogenic recessivity with complete penetrance as the primary cause of ARNSHI (Stevenson and Cheeseman, 1956; Chung et al., 1959; Fraser, 1976; Hu et al., 1987).

ARNSHI is heterogeneous, although the degree of heterogeneity is open to speculation. Hu et al. (1987) estimated that 5–6 loci cause ARNSHI in the Zhabei district of Shanghai; Chung et al. (1959) calculated the number of ARNSHI loci to be 36 from data collected in Northern Ireland; Chung and Brown (1970) studied the segregation of deaf families ascertained through the Clarke School for the Deaf in Northampton, Massachusetts, and concluded that the number of loci is 5–103; and Sank (1963) proposed the broadest range, 45–6300 loci, in a study of the genetic aspects of total deafness in the USA. In separate calculations using data provided by these investigators, Morton (1991) estimated the number of ARNSHI loci to be 4–60. The ultimate answer must be supported by the clinical delineation of these presumed loci, which is not a trivial undertaking.

Heterogeneity has made the identification of ARNSHI loci challenging for two reasons. First, single families of a size suitable for conventional linkage analysis are not common, and second, pooling of multiple small families is precluded by the inability to subclassify ARNSHI reliably by audiometric criteria (Fukushima et al., 1995a). To date (October 1997), 20 ARNSHI genes have been identified (Van Camp and Smith, 1995), although only two have been cloned (Van Camp and Smith, 1997).

Several different approaches have been used to localize ARNSHI genes. Two loci, *DFNB1* and *DFNB2*, were mapped in multiply inbred families from highly endogamous areas in Tunisia. Families with *DFNB1* originated from the northern province of Nabeul (Guilford et al., 1994a), and families with *DFNB2*, from a village 30 km from Sfax in the southern part of the country (Guilford et al., 1994b). Two additional Tunisian clusters of ARNSHI also have been reported (Ben Arab et al., 1990). The third reported locus, *DFNB3*, was mapped in an endogamous population in a remote village in Bengala, Bali. Although there were no definitely consanguineous marriages, 47 of 2185 villagers had

ARNSHI (Friedman et al., 1995). To localize this gene, Friedman et al. (1995) developed and used a method of linkage analysis known as allele-frequency-dependent homozygosity mapping. Most of the remaining loci have been identified in consanguineous nuclear families by homozygosity mapping (HM), suggesting that this strategy can be exploited to localize ARNSHI genes.

Homozygosity mapping in consanguineous families

The relationship between consanguinity and disease expression was noted by Garrod in 1902, although more than half a century passed before Smith (1953) and then Lander and Botstein (1987) explored the value of HM for mapping rare autosomal recessive diseases. HM relies on the observation that a child of a consanguineous union who is affected with a rare recessive disease is autozygous (homozygous by descent HBD) around the disease locus; a region of many centiMorgans (cM) is HBD around the disease locus in other similarly affected children born of the same union. Although additional regions of the genome are also HBD in each individual child, these regions are not constant from one affected person to the next.

The theoretical benefit this provides for disease mapping requires dense genetic maps of highly polymorphic markers and appropriate computer algorithms to analyse the generated data. Neither of these resources was available in the 1950s, forcing Smith (1953) to conclude that a HBD mapping strategy was not practical. The same limitations still existed in 1987. However, current maps (Weissenbach et al., 1992; Buetow et al., 1994; Gyapay et al., 1994) and algorithms (Kruglyak et al., 1995) are sufficient to support this research.

The value of HM to localize ARNSHI genes is predicted by segregation analyses of sibships of consanguineous unions. These analyses provide a high degree of assurance that hearing impairment in multiplex sibships is the result of monogenic recessive inheritance of fully penetrant genes without sporadic cases (Stevenson and Cheeseman, 1956; Chung et al., 1959; Morton, 1991). For each consanguineous union, the likelihood of HBD, referred to as the coefficient of inbreeding, F, varies with the marital relationship. For first-cousin marriages, $F = 1/16$, whereas for uncle–niece and second-cousin marriages, F is 1/8 and 1/64, respectively. If a disease allele that causes ARNSHI occurs with frequency q in a population in Hardy–Weinberg equilibrium, the probability, a, that an affected child is HBD at the disease locus is $Fq/[Fq+(1-F)q^2]$, where Fq of affected progeny are HBD and $(1-F)q^2$ of affected progeny are affected due to random meeting of disease alleles (Lander and Botstein, 1987). If q is small compared to F, $(1-F)q^2 < Fq$ and a approaches 1.

In a consanguineous marriage, allelic homozygosity with an infinitely polymorphic marker necessarily implies HBD around that marker. The odds ratio in favour of linkage between the marker and the ARNSHI gene, as compared to no linkage, is a/F, and the lod score, Z, obtained from a single affected child of a first-cousin marriage is $\log_{10} (a/F) = \log_{10} (16/1) = 1.2$. For four affected children of this union, $Z>3.0$, providing evidence of linkage (the first affected child establishes phase and contributes ~1.2 to the lod score; each subsequent affected child contributes ~0.6 to the lod score). In a non-consanguineous union, in contrast, a minimum of four grandparents, two parents and four affected and 12 unaffected progeny are required to obtain a lod score >3 (SLINK Monte-Carlo simulations using a polymorphic marker with six alleles and coding the ARNSHI gene as fully penetrant (Weeks et al., 1990)).

Regions of the world that deserve special attention for HM include parts of Italy, the Middle East and India (Lander and Botstein, 1987). In southern India, in particular, approximately 25% of Hindu marriages are consanguineous (Roychoudhury, 1976), most frequently between first-cousins and uncle–nieces (Roychoudhury, 1980). This population can be used to estimate the mean frequency of ARNSHI disease alleles and the number of expected loci.

Estimating the number of loci causing ARNSHI in southern India

To estimate the number of loci that cause ARNSHI in southern India, 43 consanguineous nuclear families with probable ARNSHI were ascertained by identifying probands from four schools for the deaf (St Louis Institute for the Deaf and the Blind, CSI School for the Deaf, Little Flower Covenant School for the Deaf and Bala Vidyalaya School for the Deaf) and The Institute of Basic Medical Sciences in Madras, India. Only families with prelingual severe-to-profound ARNSHI were included in this study. Data on the hearing status of each individual were gathered through repeated household visits, and audiograms were obtained to confirm severe-to-profound hearing impairment. Conditions such as rubella, prematurity, drug use during pregnancy, perinatal trauma and meningitis were eliminated by history. The biological relationship between spouses was determined by extensive questioning and verified by elderly members of the household. Nuclear families were extended if several other family members resided in the vicinity. The calculated maximal lod scores ranged from 1.51 to 8.44.

Genomic DNA from blood samples (Grimberg et al., 1989) was used to make a single test pool for each family containing equimolar amounts of DNA from each affected person (Fukushima et al., 1995a). The pool was screened for allelic homozygosity by use of three highly polymorphic markers for each of the first seven reported ARNSHI loci, and at each locus, homozygosity with at least one marker was demonstrable in several families (Table 13.1). For each of these families, additional flanking markers were typed to reconstruct haplotypes. Results were consistent with HBD in at least one family (range 1–3) at each locus, a finding consistent with linkage.

Table 13.1 Screening markers for each ARNSHI locus

Locus	Location	Screening markers	N_{DFNBi}	N_{HBD}	q
DFNB1	13q12	D13S143 D13S175 D13S292	6	2 (4.7%)	0.00074
DFNB2	11q13.5	D11S911 D11S527 D11S937	6	2 (4.7%)	0.00074
DFNB3	17p11.2–q12	D17S953 D17S805 D17S798	8	1 (2.3%)	0.00037
DFNB4	7q31	D7S501 D7S496 D7S523	6	3 (2.3%)	0.00110
DFNB5	14q12	D14S79 D14S253 D14S286	5	2 (4.7%)	0.00074
DFNB6	3p21	D3S1767 D3S1289 D3S1582	6	1 (2.3%)	0.00037
DFNB7	9q13	D9S50 D9S301 D9S166	15	3 (6.9%)	0.00110

N_{DFNBi} in which affected persons were homozygous with at least one marker (N_{total} = 43), and the number of families, N_{HBD}, in which HBD was probable based on haplotype reconstruction (q = calculated gene frequency for each locus in Tamil Nadu). PCR-amplification of polymorphic markers was performed using 30-ng DNA template and 1 μl of each primer (10 μM). Sequences for primer pairs are listed in the Genome Database (GDB). DNA was denatured for 30 s at 95°C, annealed with PCR primers at 55°C for 30 s, and extended with 1 unit of *Taq* DNA polymerase (Amersham) at 72°C for 30 s for a total of 25 cycles, followed by a post-PCR extension step at 72°C for 10 min. Polymerase buffer as supplied by the vendor was used and supplemented with 1 μl each of 10 mM dATP, dTTP, and dGTP. Radioactive I^{32}PdCTP (1 μl) was added with 1 μl unlabelled dCTP (0.1 mM). Reaction products were resolved on a 6% polyacrylamide gel, followed by drying and autoradiography. With some primer pairs, reaction conditions were modified to optimize amplification.

To estimate the number of ARNSHI genes, the mean value, q, of the frequency of genes that cause ARNSHI in a given population must be calculated. In general, the frequency of deafness, D_i, caused by the ith deafness gene is $D_i = Fq_i + (1-F)q_i^2$, where F is the inbreeding coefficient in the particular population and qi is the gene frequency of the ith deafness gene. Expressed in terms of q_i, $q_i = \{-F + [F^2 + 4D_i(1-F)]^{0.5}\}/[2(1-F)]$ (Morton,

1991). Reported values for q range widely (Morton, 1991) and all have been estimated without knowing the frequency of any ARNSHI genes.

In the rural area of Tamil Nadu, F and $D = \sum D_i$ are estimated to be 0.0371 (Rao and Inbaraj, 1980) and 0.0006 (Majumder et al., 1989), respectively. Based on these values, the frequency of each of the first seven ARNSHI genes can be calculated from the contribution ratio of each deafness locus by family as $D_{DFNBi} = (0.0006 \times n_{DFBNi})/43$, where n_{DFNBi} is the number of families mapping to that locus. For *DFNB5*, for example, $D_{DFNB5} = (0.0006 \ x2)/43 = 0.000014$ and $q_{DFNB5} = 0.00074$ (see Table 13.1 above). Based on the panmictic (A) and inbred (B) loads of this population (0.044 and 0.00015, respectively (Morton, 1991)), and the mean gene frequency, q, calculated from the gene frequencies for *DFNB1-7* ($[q_{DFNB1} + \ldots + q_{DFNB7}]/7$), the number of ARNSHI loci, k, can be estimated: $k = (A + B)/q = (0.044 + 0.00015)/0.00075 = 57$. This calculation assumes that HBD implies linkage to the particular locus being studied.

The power of a specific number of consanguineous multiplex families to localise ARNSHL genes can be determined from simulations of the sampling distribution of 57 loci performed using the prevalence values for *DFNB1-7* shown in Table 13.1 above and a mean prevalence of 0.013 ($29/[43 \times 50]$) for the remaining loci (10 000 simulations, SAS Uniform Random Number Generator). With 50 multiplex families, 27-34 loci can be identified with 90% probability (Table 13.2). If the number of families is increased to 200, the range of loci that can be identified increases to 51-56. To identify all loci with 90% probability, 357 families must be tested.

Table 13.2 Expected number of ARNSHI genes that could be identified with 90% probability as a function of the number of consanguineous nuclear familes tested. The calculation assumes equal frequencies of all genes except *DFNB1-7*.

Families	ARNSHI loci
50	27-34
100	40-47
150	47-53
200	51-56

Possible digenic inheritance in ARNSHI

The validity of HM to localize ARNSHI genes is supported by estimates of the segregation frequency of deafness, p, in non-consanguineous and consanguineous marriages. In non-consanguineous marriages, p is very close to 0.25 (0.228-0.27), allowing for a proportion of sporadic cases of hearing loss due to:

• Unrecognized acquired causes.
• Dominant, sex-linked or mitochondrial mutations.
• Complex inheritance patterns with low recurrence risk.

This result is consistent with monogenic recessivity and complete penetrance (Chung et al., 1959; Sank, 1963; Chung and Brown, 1970; Ben Arab et al., 1990).

In consanguineous unions, p also approximates 0.25, implying that more complex genetic mechanisms are rare (Kimberling et al., 1989). However, Majumder et al. (1989) have presented data to suggest that the most parsimonious model for ARNSHI involves paired unlinked diallelic autosomal loci. With this theory individuals are hearing impaired only if they are recessively homozygous at both loci.

Polygenic inheritance has been reported in several other diseases. Retinitis pigmentosa (RP), a genetically heterogenous disease usually inherited in a simple autosomal dominant or recessive manner, can also be caused by co-inheritance of specific mutations at the unlinked peripherin/RDS and ROM1 loci on chromosomes 6p and 11q, respectively (Kajiwara et al., 1994). Heterozygotes for either the peripherin/RDS or ROM1 mutations alone have electroretinograms similar to recessive RP carriers, but only combined heterozygotes for both genes show the clinical phenotype.

In mice, an extreme form of spina bifida that resembles spina bifida occulta in humans has been reported in *undulated-Patch* double-mutant mice (Helwig et al., 1995), and other doubly mutant animals have been reported that are highly susceptible to infections (Froidevaux and Loor, 1991; Lowell et al., 1994). The development of overt diabetes in nonobese diabetic mice is even more complex and requires homozygosity for at least three recessive genes (Prochazka et al., 1987).

Digenic inheritance of ARNSHI has not been reported. Interestingly, we have identified a small consanguineous family in which this is a possibility (first-cousin marriage with three affected and three non-affected progeny). Two genomic DNA pools, one from the affected children and the other from their siblings and the parents, were used to screen 165 short tandem repeat polymorphic markers (STRPs) evenly spaced across the autosomal human genome. PCR products were resolved on 6% denaturing polyacrylamide gels by silver staining. With nine STRPs, a single allele in the affected sibling pool was associated with two or three alleles in the non-affected pool, and with 14 STRPs, a single common allele was observed in both DNA pools. By typing flanking markers and reconstructing haplotypes, HBD was eliminated in 20 cases, but not for three STRPs (GATA4A10 and GATA3CO2 on chromosome 3 and D19S216 on chromosome 19). Additional STRPs confirmed HBD over a 39 cM region on chromosome 3 and a 32 cM region on chromosome 19 (Tables 13.3 and 13.4). Lod scores over both intervals are equal at −2.79.

Table 13.3 Allele frequencies for chromosome 3 STRPs showing HBD in family used to localize *DFNB15*

STRP	Size (bp)	Allele frequency
D3S1764	234	0.174
D3S1576	189	0.158
D3S1316	276	0.097
D3S1309	133	0.029
D3S1550	143	0.184
D3S1593	134	0.131
D3S1557	198	0.250
D3S1744	157	0.068
D3S1306	156	0.054
D3S1555	220	0.329
D3S1308	93	0.329
D3S1279	272	0.341
D3S1315	239	0.081
D3S1237	193	0.184
D3S1584	158	0.181
GATA8FO1	247	0.051
D3S1275	254	0.108
D3S1605	146	0.092
D3S1607	228	0.308
D3S1553	172	0.579
D3S1268	120	0.043
D3S1258	175	0.053

Calculations based on data from 40 unrelated persons from the same geographic area and of the same ethnic origin: allele frequencies used to calculate lod score of 2.79

Table 13.4 Allele frequencies for chromosome 19 STRPs showing HBD family used to localize *DFNB15*

STRP	Size (bp)	Allele frequency
D19S209	272	0.421
D19S424	147	0.181
D19S591	103	0.309
D19S177	167	0.444
D19S216	190	0.182
D19S427	118	0.069
D19S406	214	0.014
INSR	137	0.069
D19S592	266	0.278
D19S1034	232	0.216
D19S413	118	0.182
D19S221	154	0.085
D19S226	255	0.044
D19S411	157	0.014

Calculations based on data from 40 unrelated persons from the same geographic area and of the same ethnic origin: allele frequencies used to calculate lod score of 2.79

These regions each offer intriguing possibilities as a new DFNB locus. The interval flanked by *D3S1290* and *D3S1282* on chromosome 3q21.3–q25.2 includes the gene for Usher syndrome type III (*USH3*) (Sankila et al., 1995) and suggests that these two types of deafness may be allelic. This possibility is made more attractive by the association of *USH1B* (Kimberling et al., 1990; Smith et al., 1992) with *DFNB2* (Guilford et al., 1994b) and *DFNA11* (Tamagawa et al., 1996), and *USH1D* (Wayne et al., 1997) with *DFNB12* (Chaib et al., 1996). Although the *DFNA11*, *DFNB12* and *USH1D* genes have not been cloned, *USH1B* and *DFNB2* are both caused by mutations in an unconventional myosin, MYOVIIA (Liu et al., 1997; Weil et al., 1995 and 1997).

Based on mouse homologies to human chromosome 3, possible animal models include the *flaky tail* (*ft*), *deafwaddler* (*dfw*), and *spinner* (*sr*) mutants. The *flaky tail* gene (mouse chromosome 3, cM position 41.4) is expressed in homozygotes as a phenotype characterized by the stretched appearance of skin over the feet and hands, early constriction of the tail and pinnae and hearing defects (Lane, 1972). By day-of-life 14, the flakiness disappears and with the exception of small ears and an occasional amputated tail, *ft/ft* mice appear normal. The *deafwaddler* gene is on distal mouse chromosome 6 in an area that shows homology to human chromosomes 12p and 3q21–q24 (Street et al., 1995). Homozygotes walk with a hesitant and wobbly gait, display head bobbing, and are deaf secondary to progressive degeneration of cochlear hair cells (Lane, 1987). The *spinner* gene is on chromosome 9 and is flanked by genes that map to human chromosome 3p22–p21.3 and 3q23–q25. Homozygotes show the typical head tossing, circling, deafness and hyperactivity of shaker–waltzer mutants. Inner ear anomalies include degeneration of the organ of Corti and spiral ganglion, reduction in size of the stria vascularis, and limited degeneration of the saccular macula (Deol and Robins, 1962).

The interval flanked by *D19S424* and *D19S415* on chromosome 19p13.3–p13.1 includes two genes that may be important for normal auditory function. The first, *MYO1F*, is an unconventional myosin (Hasson et al., 1996). Although its expression in the inner ear has not been studied, three other unconventional myosins, *MYO1C*, *MYO6* and *MYOVIIA*, do play important roles in hair cell architecture and function (Hasson et al., 1996). The *MYO1C* and *MYO6* loci have not been linked to any types of hereditary hearing impairment but, as previously mentioned, mutations in *MYOVIIA* have been demonstrated in *USH1B* (Weil et al., 1995) and *DFNB2* (Liu et al., 1997; Weil et al., 1997).

The second gene, *Notch*, encodes a signal receptor in *Drosophila* that acts with two ligands, *Delta* and *Serrate*, to control cell fate through a process of lateral inhibition (Heitzler and Simpson, 1991). If a cell receives a signal from *Delta*, it becomes committed to a specific pathway and inhibits its neighbours from doing the same; ectopic expression of *Serrate* rescues *Delta* mutants (Gu et al., 1995). The importance of this type of cell–cell signalling in the inner ear is suggested by its striking pattern of differentiation (Goodyear et al., 1994). Although a functional role of the three mammalian homologues of *Notch* has not been determined and evidence is only circumstantial, avian homologues of *Notch*, *Delta* and *Serrate* are expressed early in ear development (Myat et al., 1996).

Based on mouse homologies to human chromosome 19, a possible animal model is the *mocha* (*mh*) mutant. Homozygote *mh/mh* mice exhibit postnatal cochlear degeneration (Lane and Deol, 1974). Abnormal auditory brainstem responses are demonstrable at 2 weeks of age and disappear by 6 months of age (Rolfsen and Erway, 1984).

These data identify one of these chromosomal regions as the site of a new locus for ARNSHI; however the possibility of digenic recessive inheritance must also be considered. Although definitive proof must await gene cloning, additional families with a similar genotype would strongly suggest that digenic recessive inheritance can lead to ARNSHI.

Homozygosity mapping applied to Usher syndrome

Deaf-blindness in humans is most frequently caused by the Usher syndromes (USH), a group of disorders characterized by autosomal recessive inheritance and dual sensory impairments. Affected individuals have sensorineural hearing loss and become visually impaired secondary to progressive pigmentary retinopathy (PPR) (Smith et al., 1994). To date, three phenotypically distinct forms of USH have been described and mapped to six different genomic regions (Table 13.5).

At least one additional USH gene exists: a few families with Ush1 have been identified that do not map to any of the reported USH loci, and nearly 10% of Ush2 families have been excluded from chromosome 1q. The absence of a sufficient number of unmapped families and the possibility of further heterogeneity preclude identification of new loci by classical linkage analysis. However, a first-cousin marriage that has produced four children with the clinical diagnosis of Ush1 has been used to identify a fourth locus, *USH1D* (Wayne et al., 1997).

After excluding linkage to known USH loci (Table 13.5), two genomic DNA pools, one from the affected children and the other from the parents, were used to screen 161 highly polymorphic markers evenly spaced across the autosomal human genome. Seven shifts to allelic homozygosity were observed in the affected sibling pool and evaluated by typing closely linked flanking markers and reconstructing haplotypes. The only autosomal region showing HBD flanked *GATA87G01*. Based on consistent allelic homozygosity, a 15 cM region bounded by *D10S529* and *D10S573* was identified as the location of the *USH1D* gene. Lod scores calculated using MAPMAKER/HOMOZ

Table 13.5 Phenotypic and genotypic data for the Usher syndromes

Usher type	Phenotype	Chromosome	Gene	Screening markers
Ush1	Congenital severe to profound hearing loss; absent vestibular function; PPR	USH1A–14q (Kaplan et al., 1992)	Myosin VIIA	D14S267, D14S250, D14S78
		USH1B–11q (Kimberling et al., 1992)	?	D11S911, D11S527, D11S937
		USH1C–11p (Smith et al., 1992)	?	D11S902, D11S921, D11S1888
		USH1D–10q (Wayne et al., 1997)	?	D10S529, D10S202, D10S572
		USH1E–21q (Chaib et al., 1997)	?	D21S1884,D21S1257,
				D21S265, D21S1258
		USH1F–10 (Wayne et al., 1997)	?	D10S199, D10S578, D10S596
Ush2	Congenital moderate to severe hearing loss; normal vestibular function; PPR	USH2A–1q (Kimberling et al., 1990)	?	D1S237, D1S474, D1S229
Ush3	Congenital moderate to severe hearing loss; normal vestibular function; PR	3p (Sankila et al., 1995)	?	D3S1308, D3S1299, D3S1279

(Kruglyak et al., 1995) confirm this linkage (Z=~3.0). This region also is the site of *DFNB11*.

Comparative human–mouse mapping suggests that *Jackson circler* (*Jc*), *waltzer* (*v*), or *Ames waltzer* (*Av*) may represent the mouse model of *USH1D*. Each of these mutants is recessive and shows the typical circling, head-tossing, and hyperactive behaviour associated with deafness and vestibular dysfunction (Lyon and Searle, 1989). Although Jc has not been studied for inner ear anomalies, in the other two mouse mutants, degenerative changes of the membranous labyrinth have been described (Deol, 1956; Kocher, 1960; Osako and Hilding, 1971). None has any reported retinal pathology. However it is worth noting that *shaker-1* (*sh-1*), the mouse model of *USH1B*, also has no evidence of pigmentary retinopathy (Gibson et al., 1995). Interestingly, *Waltzer–shaker-1* double heterozygotes (*v/+ sh-1/+*) become deaf at age 3–6 months and have changes similar to *v/v* homozygotes in the organ of Corti, stria vascularis, and spiral ganglion (Kocher, 1960; Osako and Hilding, 1971). This phenotype suggests an interaction between myosinVIIA and the *waltzer* gene, making the latter a strong candidate for the *USH1D* gene.

Limitations of homozygosity mapping as applied to ARNSHI and USH

Classically, once a specific chromosome has been identified, the minimal size of the interval that contains the disease gene is established by expanding the family to include as many individuals as possible, reconstructing haplotypes to identify recombination events, and typing additional markers in informative individuals to narrow the crossover interval. Including other presumably genotypically identical families is usually of enormous benefit. Unfortunately, although heterogeneity and consanguinity facilitate gene localisation, they are serious drawbacks to gene cloning. Additional genotypically similar families with ARNSHI and USH1D are difficult to identify and consanguinity produces large regions of HBD. Flanking markers, therefore, are often 20–30 cM apart.

Contiguous physical maps of this size are very time-consuming to construct and screen for coding sequence. Since our ultimate goal is to have an effect on healthcare and habilitation for the hearing impaired, the most frequently occurring deafness genes are the most biologically relevant and should be cloned first. Other important considerations include the existence of murine homologues, the possibility of allelic mutations producing other deafness phenotypes, and the size of the candidate interval. On these bases, *DFNB1*, *DFNB4* and *DFNB7* should be cloned first.

Conclusions

HM is a powerful strategy for localizing genes that cause autosomal recessive non-syndromic hearing impairment (ARNSHI) and rare types of syndromal hearing impairment (SHI). Regions of the world that deserve special attention for HM include parts of Italy, the Middle East and India (Lander and Botstein, 1987). In southern India, in particular, approximately 25% of Hindu marriages are consanguineous (Roychoudhury, 1976), most frequently between first cousins and uncle–nieces (Roychoudhury, 1980).

In this study, consanguineous families with two or more progeny with ARNSHI were ascertained in southern India and used to estimate the mean frequency of ARNSHI disease alleles and to calculate the number of disease loci (57). In one family, digenic recessive inheritance appears possible. A first-cousin marriage that produced four children with the clinical diagnosis of Ush1 also was used to identify a fourth locus, Ush1D (Wayne et al., 1997).

Acknowledgements

This work was supported in part by research grant numbers 1RO1 DC02046 and 1RO1 DC02842 from the National Institute on Deafness and Other Communication Disorders, National Institutes of Health (RJHS).

Chapter 14
A Turkish kindred with autosomal recessive non-syndromal hearing impairment segregates *DFNB9*

SM LEAL, E VITALE, F APAYDIN, Y HU, C BARNWELL,
M IBER, T KANDOGAN, U BRAENDLE, HP ZENNER,
M SCHWALB and O CURA

Abstract

The autosomal recessive sensorineural hearing loss gene *DFNB9* was previously mapped to 2p22–23 in a consanguineous family from Lebanon. We have evidence that an additional autosomal recessive non-syndromal hearing impairment (ARNSHI) kindred segregates *DFNB9*. Linkage was established to markers closely linked to *DFNB9* in a consanguineous kindred from eastern Turkey. A maximum lod score of 3.4 was obtained for *D2S174* which lies within the 2cM support region for *DFNB9*.

This kindred, Turkey-21 is highly consanguineous with four affected members, two of whom are siblings. All affected individuals are the offspring of consanguineous matings. The hearing loss for affected individuals within this kindred is profound with onset diagnosed before the second year of life.

Two additional consanguineous ARNSHI kindreds from western Turkey were genotyped for markers closely linked to *DFNB9*. Linkage was excluded from the genetic region of *DFNB9* for each of these kindreds. One of these kindreds, Turkey-22, which is highly consanguineous can independently establish linkage. This kindred was tested for linkage to all known ARNSHI loci. A complete genome scan will be used to localize the non-syndromal hearing impairment (NSHI) locus segregating in this kindred.

To date, 52 NSHI pedigrees with two or more affected individuals have been identified in Turkey. From this group of pedigrees the following modes of inheritance are exhibited: three autosomal dominant; 17 autosomal recessive (12 of these kindreds contain at least one consanguineous mating); five X-linked; and 27 with unknown aetiology. Simulation analysis demonstrated that six of these kindreds can establish linkage independently: X-linked NSHI kindreds, Turkey-2 (ELOD 2.2; power 0.6), and Turkey-9 (ELOD 2.0; power 0.8); autosomal dominant Turkey-3 (ELOD 3.23; power 0.65) and Turkey-4 (ELOD 2.62; power 0.45); and autosomal recessive Turkey-21 (ELOD 3.07; power 0.6) and Turkey-22 (ELOD 3.90; power 0.9).

Chapter 15

Assessment of the contribution of the loci *DFNA1–10* and *DFNB1–9* in inherited hearing impairment in two populations: the United Arab Emirates and the British Pakistani populations

KA BROWN, G KARBANI, G PARRY, LL MOYNIHAN,
AH JANJUA, LI AL-GAZALI, VE NEWTON, AF MARKHAM and
RF MUELLER

Abstract

Ten loci for autosomal dominant hearing impairment (*DFNA1–10*) and nine loci for autosomal recessive (*DFNB1–9*) hearing loss have recently been identified, the latter in a number of genetically isolated populations by autozygosity mapping. Each genetically isolated population can be expected to have a unique subset of genes involved in hearing impairment. However, a number of the genes in that subset will also be involved in hearing impairment in other populations. In addition, loci implicated in dominant hearing loss in one population may contribute to recessive forms of hearing loss in other populations. To compare the relative frequencies of the known hearing impairment loci in two populations of interest autozygosity mapping were used to analyse 27 consanguineous families from the British population originating from the Mirpur region of Pakistan and 12 consanguineous families from the United Arab Emirates (UAE), all of which segregate non-syndromal autosomal recessive hearing impairment.

Preliminary data suggest that the UAE population segregates the recessive loci *DFNB4*, *DFNB8* and *DFNB9*, with one family apparently linked in each case, whilst the British Pakistani population segregates the loci *DFNB1*, *DFNB3*, *DFNB4* and *DFNB5* with four, one, three and one families, respectively, potentially linked in each instance. The two populations therefore appear to segregate different combinations of the known recessive hearing loss loci. In addition, loci originally described in families with dominantly inherited forms of hearing impairment are implicated in autosomal recessive hearing impairment in both populations; *DFNA2* and *DFNA8* in one and two families, respectively, from the UAE and *DFNA5* in one family from the British Pakistani population.

PART VII
NON-SYNDROMAL AUTOSOMAL DOMINANT HEARING IMPAIRMENT

Chapter 16
Hereditary dominant non-syndromal progressive hearing impairment in a large family in southern Italy

A BOJANO, L CALIFANO and P CAPPARUCCIA

Introduction

Genetic hearing impairments occur in isolated forms (non-syndromal) in 70% of cases and are associated with other disorders (syndromal) in 30% (Gorlin et al., 1995).

Genetic research carried out in families with non-syndromal hearing impairment (NSHI) has shown considerable heterogeneity, comprising at least 10 different mutations both for the dominant (DFNA) and for the recessive (DFNB) form (Tranebjaerg, 1996). It is this genetic hetero-geneity which complicates gene mapping by linkage analysis (Martini et al., 1996). Research on dominant NSHI has so far indicated over eight mutations, located in chromosomes 1, 4, 5, 7, 13, 15 and 19 (Dallapiccola et al., 1996a).

Family

A study was made of a large family (Figure 16.1) with non-syndromal dominantly inherited autosomal hearing impairment with high pene-trance comprising five generations with 52 members, 52% of whom (27

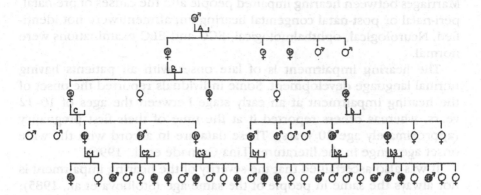

Figure 16.1 The family.

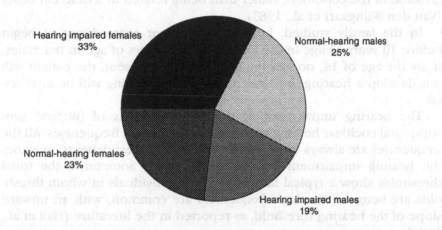

Figure 16.2 The relatives: breakdown of normally hearing and hearing impaired males and females.

individuals) show hearing impairment (Figure 16.2). Thirty-seven per cent of the affected group were males and 63% females.

There is also a sixth generation, comprising 28 people (15 M; 13 F). Even though three affected members were detected, in addition to a male with Down syndrome, this generation was not included in the results of the research as it consists mainly of children in many of whom the disease has not yet had time to reveal itself.

The transmission of hearing impairment does not undergo a generation gap; it is always present and only appears in the offspring of affected parents. No relationship was found between the patient's sex and the hearing impairment.

The anamnesis carried out in all screened patients allowed other pathologies associated with hearing impairment to be excluded, as well as consanguineous marriages, at least in the generations still alive.

Marriages between hearing impaired people and the causes of pre-natal, peri-natal or post-natal congenital hearing impairment were not identified. Neurological, ophthalmological, ECG and EEG examinations were normal.

The hearing impairment is of late onset with all patients having normal language development. Some individuals reported the onset of the hearing impairment at an early stage between the ages of 10–12 years, whereas others reported it at the time of their first pregnancy (approximately age 20 years). These data are in accord with the wide onset age range in the literature. (Lina-Granade et al., 1996).

It was also ascertained that the severity of the hearing impairment is not always the same in people of the same age (Stolbova et al., 1985); tonal thresholds of patients of the same age sometimes showed 40 dB differences. This was found to be due to individual variability in the progression of the condition, rather than being related to a different onset (Van den Wijngaart et al., 1985).

In the family studied, hearing impairment seemed not to begin before 10 years of age in the females and 12 years of age in the males. If, by the age of 14, no hearing impairment is present, the patient will not develop a hearing impairment and their offspring will be unaffected.

The hearing impairment of the family consists of bilateral sensorineural cochlear hearing impairment affecting all frequencies. All the frequencies are always involved, even in the youngest patients, in whom the hearing impairment was of recent onset. Sometimes the tonal thresholds show a typical flat pattern, but individuals in whom thresholds are better at the high frequencies are common, with an upward slope of the hearing threshold, as reported in the literature (Hall et al., 1996).

In some cases a more severe involvement was found in the mid-frequencies with saucer-shaped thresholds (Figure 16.3).

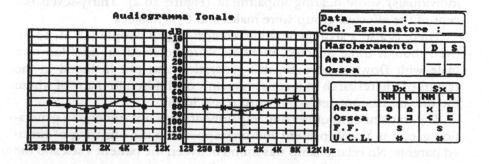

Figure 16.3 Family branch C³, No. 5, 17 years old.

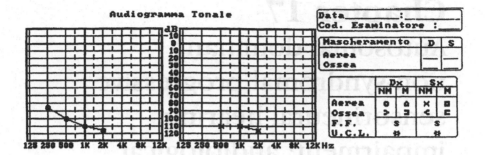

Figure 16.4 Family branch C, No. 5, 50 years old.

In middle-aged patients, who had a severe hearing impairment, flat thresholds were found, although in some people there is no measurable high-frequency hearing. In the more advanced cases, there is only residual hearing in the mid and low frequencies (Figure 16.4), with deterioration of their speech and language.

Detailed study of this family indicated some psychological problems. Many reacted to their hearing impairment in an adverse way. The feeling of shame added to the onset of the hearing impairment leading to the concept of an inevitable punishment for which medical science could do nothing, made many relatives paranoid. They often refused to have careful audiological, biochemical, haematological and genetic analyses and also refused these for their normally hearing children. Many purchased hearing aids independently, avoiding specialist clinical examination.

We consider that the study of a family suffering from genetic hearing impairment requires the following steps:

- Provision of periodic audiological check-ups for the largest number of relatives possible.
- Genetic mapping.
- Provision of information about the risks of the children of affected parents, especially in families who show a high penetrance.
- Consideration of ways of reducing the disability and handicap in the long term, by encouraging early hearing aid use by the affected patients.
- Analysis of the younger relatives, to detect the onset of hearing impairment at an earlier stage.
- Formation of a collaborative team, including audiologists, psychologists, geneticists and hearing aid technicians.

Chapter 17
Autosomal dominant non-syndromal progressive sensorineural hearing impairment: audiological evaluation of a Dutch *DFNA2* family

H KUNST, HAM MARRES, PLM HUYGEN, P COUCKE,
P WILLEMS and CWRJ CREMERS

Abstract

A large Dutch family with a pedigree spanning six generations, who showed a hereditary trait of non-syndromal sensorineural hearing impairment (ADNSHI) is presented. Linkage to the *DFNA2* locus could be obtained in affected individuals. We give a description of the phenotype of this *DFNA2*-linked family.

In a linear regression analysis of individual hearing thresholds (most recent audiogram) on age, significant progression was found at all frequencies, but the onset threshold was higher at the high frequencies (around 30 dB at 2–8 kHz) than at the lower ones (around 0 dB at 0.25–1 kHz). It is possible that some hearing impairment is present at the higher frequencies at birth or in early childhood. The regression coefficient, or the 'annual threshold increase' (ATI), expressed in dB/year, was about 1 dB/year on average, but the higher frequencies (1–8 kHz) showed significantly more rapid progression (ATI 1.03–1.11 dB/year) than the lower frequencies (0.25–0.5 kHz; ATI 0.88–0.89 dB/year). The age at which an affected person will require a hearing aid is estimated at between 10–50 years. Remarkably, the clinical presentation and the natural history of ADNSHI in the present family was completely similar to another unrelated Dutch family with linkage to the same *DFNA2* region.

Some typical audiograms are presented in Figure 17.1. There was a large intrafamilial variation in features and in the progression of the hearing impairment. A 95% range for the ATI of approximately 0.6–1.3 dB/year was calculated. This explains the wide range of ages at which a hearing aid will be needed. In Figure 17.1 the mean threshold of all 26 genetically affected persons is depicted as a grey band. Note the shift in threshold from below to above the mean threshold as age increases.

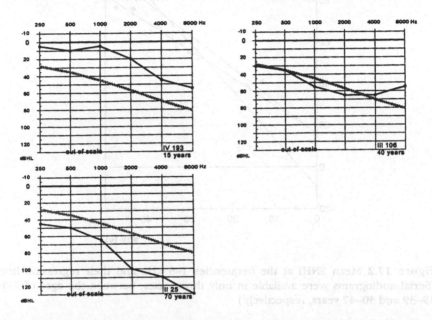

Figure 17.1 Three cases, one each from generations IV, III and II exemplifying the initial, intermediate and final stages of (progressive) hearing impairment, respectively (left ear). The mean audiogram (corresponding to a mean age of 38 years) of all 26 cases is shown as a grey band.

Sufficient longitudinal data for regression analysis of threshold data were available in only three cases: Figure 17.2 shows the mean threshold for the frequencies 1–8 kHz. There was no strong indication of any non-linearity in the hearing impairment, such as, for example, onset after birth and excessive progression during the first few years after onset. The individual regression lines in Figure 17.2 showed more variability than the group regression lines, presumably because of the smaller number of observations. Individual ATI values for the longitudinal data were in the range of 0.2–2.3 dB/year, i.e. up to higher values than those derived for the group statistics from the most recent audiogram. The ATI at the higher frequencies was greater than that at the lower frequencies.

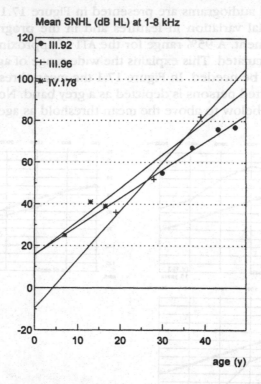

Figure 17.2 Mean SNHI at the frequencies 1–8 kHz and their regression lines. (Serial audiograms were available in only three cases, between the ages of 7–16, 19–39 and 30–47 years, respectively.)

The variability and the degree of progression in these three cases seemed to be rather excessive, even allowing for the small number of observations. We have no doubt that these three cases must have presented for serial audiometry because of the pronounced progression of their ADNSHI and, therefore, represent a sample of cases selected on the basis of such progression.

Chapter 18
Autosomal dominant congenital severe sensorineural hearing impairment — localization of a disease gene to chromosome 11q by linkage in an Austrian family

K KIRSCHOFER, JB KENYON, DM HOOVER, P FRANZ,
K WEIPOLTSHAMMER, F WACHTLER and WJ KIMBERLING

Abstract

In a rural region in Austria a four-generation family was found suffering from a severe, congenital non-progressive and non-syndromic sensorineural hearing impairment, showing autosomal dominant inheritance. The affected individuals showed moderate to profound sensorineural hearing loss of 60–80 dB, normal caloric vestibular responses and almost no variation from one person to another. Blood was obtained from all available members of this family, DNA was extracted and a genome search was performed using standard methods. We had a lod score of over 2.0 with markers on chromosome 15. However, haplotype analysis revealed an inconsistency in the placement of the gene. A fuller genome search was performed and revealed several positive 2-point lod scores on the long arm of chromosome 11. The highest value was 3.6, which was seen with the marker *D11S934*. Haplotype analysis excluded the gene from the chromosome proximal *D11S911* and distal to *D11S968*. These results place the gene in region overlapping with the region containing *DFNA12*, *DFNA11* and *DFNA12*, respectively.

PART VIII
X-LINKED HEARING IMPAIRMENT

Chapter 19
Identification of a novel locus for non-syndromal X-linked sensorineural hearing impairment (*DFN6*) on Xp22

I DEL CASTILLO, M VILLAMAR, M SARDUY, L ROMERO, C HERRAIZ, FJ HERNANDEZ, M RODRIGUEZ, I BORRAS, A MONTERO, J BELLON, MC TAPIA and F MORENO

Abstract

Non-syndromal X-linked hearing impairment is highly heterogenous. At least five different clinical forms have been described, but only two loci have been mapped. A Spanish family affected by a previously undescribed X-linked form of hearing impairment was studied. In this family, hearing impairment is non-syndromal, sensorineural and progressive. The auditory impairment in affected males is first detected at school age and mainly involves the high frequencies. Later it evolves to become severe to profound, affecting all frequencies by adulthood. Carrier females manifest a moderate hearing impairment in the high frequencies, with the onset delayed to the fourth decade of life. Hearing impairment was assumed to be X-linked dominant, with incomplete penetrance and variable expressivity in carrier females. The family was genotyped for a set of microsatellite markers evenly spaced at intervals of about 10 cM on the X chromosome. Evidence was found of linkage to markers in the Xp22 region (maximum lod score of 5.30 at $\theta = 0.000$

for *DXS8036* and for *DXS8022*). The position of this novel hearing impairment locus (*DFN6*) was narrowed down by haplotype analysis. Mapping the breakpoints in two critical recombinants allowed the definition of an interval for *DFN6*, delimited by *DXS7108* on the distal side and by *DXS7105* on the proximal side. This critical interval spans a genetic distance of about 15 cM.

PART IX
MITOCHONDRIAL HEARING IMPAIRMENT

Chapter 20
Nuclear candidate genes for 'mitochondrial deafness'

HT JACOBS, ZH SHAH, V MIGLIOSI, SK LEHTINEN, A ROVIO
and K O'DELL

Introduction

Mitochondrial DNA (mtDNA) mutations have been implicated in both syndromal and non-syndromal sensorineural hearing impairment (SNHI) in a large number of studies. The classes of mutation which can contribute to this phenotype appear to be extremely diverse, and in no case is there any clear mechanistic understanding of how particular mutations result in the specific pathological feature of hearing impairment. In this chapter we put forward a hypothesis which attempts to relate mitochondrial genotype to the phenotype of impaired hearing, and which makes clear predictions regarding the involvement of an important new class of nuclear genes in this disorder.

Mitochondrial mutations affecting auditory function

Some of the major mitochondrial mutations that can contribute to hearing impairment are summarized in Table 20.1. At first sight, the information shown appears to have no obvious pattern. The variable tissue-specificity of mitochondrial disease phenotype is, in general terms, not understood (Wallace, 1992). It must be remembered that mtDNA encodes only a small subset of the polypeptides required for respiratory electron transfer and oxidative phosphorylation, plus the RNA components of the mitochondrial translational apparatus required for the synthesis of these few polypeptides inside mitochondria (Chomyn et al., 1987). Some specific tissues, e.g. heart and skeletal muscle and the CNS, are highly dependent on respiratory ATP generation and hence would be expected to suffer as a result of any mtDNA mutation that resulted in a generalized bioenergy deficit. However, while some mutations affecting the auditory system also affect these tissues, amongst others, other SNHI-associated mutations do not. Conversely, some mitochondrial mutations which have been shown to result in impaired respiratory metabolism, such as those in the ND1 and ND4 subunit genes associated with Leber's hereditary optic neuropathy (Wallace et al., 1988; Huoponen et al., 1991), do not affect hearing. Thus the explanation for how mtDNA mutations result in hearing impairment cannot be related simply to bioenergetic impairment. We are forced to consider the tissue-restricted involvement of nuclear genes, both for the respiratory chain and for the mitochondrial gene expression apparatus.

An important possible clue, indicating where our search should be directed, emerges from a consideration of the known or predicted effects of the various SNHI-associated mutations on mitochondrial protein metabolism. Most informative in this regard is the np 1555 mutation in the small subunit rRNA. This affects a domain of the ribosome whose function is highly conserved in evolution and which is relatively well understood (Alksne et al., 1993). Mutations in this same region of small subunit rRNA, in both bacteria and chloroplasts, affect translational accuracy. Notably, these mutations influence the susceptibility of the ribosome to aminoglycoside antibiotics, such as streptomycin, which interact with this domain to promote translational infidelity. Bacterial or chloroplast mutations in this rRNA domain fall into various classes, depending on whether they mimic or suppress other mutations in the ribosome accuracy centre which alter aminoglycoside-sensitivity. The np 1555 mutation clearly interacts with aminoglycosides in causing SNHI in humans (Prezant et al., 1993), strongly suggesting that, mechanistically, it acts by relaxing the stringency of mitochondrial protein synthesis, just like the analogous mutations in bacteria. Interestingly, the requirement for aminoglycoside involvement does not apply to all pedigrees with the np 1555 mutation, a point to which we will return later.

Interference with translational accuracy, leading to accumulation of abnormal mitochondrial translation products, is an attractive unifying hypothesis linking mtDNA mutations and SNHI, because it is supported by data gathered on at least three other mutations or mutation classes. The np 8344 point mutation in the tRNA-lys gene, associated with the MERRF syndrome, causes a defect in aminoacylation of the affected tRNA (Enriquez et al., 1995). This results in impaired translation, with documented synthesis of prematurely terminated mitochondrial translation products. The mRNAs most affected are those with the greatest number of lysine codons, suggesting that a deficiency of aminoacylated tRNA-lys underlies the effect. Although it is somewhat unclear from the literature whether SNHI is a universal feature of MERRF, the molecular observations are clearly compatible with the hypothesis put forward.

Table 20.1 Mitochondrial mutations and hearing impairment

Class of mutation	Map location (np)	Affected genes	Phenotype	Citation
Homoplasmic point mutation	1555	SSU (12S) rRNA	Hearing loss (aminoglycoside-induced in some pedigrees)	Prezant et al. (1993)
Homo- or heteroplasmic point mutation	7445	tRNA–ser (UCN)	Hearing loss	Reid et al. (1994)
Heteroplasmic point mutation	7472	tRNA–ser (UCN)	HAM syndrome (hearing loss, ataxia and myoclonus)	Tiranti et al. (1995)
Heteroplasmic point mutation	3243	tRNA–leu (UUR)	MELAS syndrome or diabetes + deafness or ocular myopathy	Van den Ouweland et al. (1992); Jean-François et al. (1994)
Heteroplasmic point mutation	8344	tRNA-lys	MERRF syndrome	Shoffner et al. (1990)
Large (>1 kb) heteroplasmic deletion	Various	Various	Ocular myopathy or Kearns–Sayre syndrome	Holt et al. (1988)
Large (>1 kb) heteroplasmic partial duplication	Various	Various	Kearns–Sayre syndrome or diabetes + deafness	Dunbar et al. (1993); Poulton et al. (1995)

Only the major, reported mutations are listed. In general, causal involvement is assumed when the mutation is absent from control pedigrees, is present in more than one affected pedigree, and where it is predicted to affect the function of at least one phylogenetically conserved nucleotide pair. Only one or two citations are given for each mutation, due to space constraints.

The np 3243 tRNA-leu(UUR) mutation is associated with a rather variable phenotype that usually includes hearing impairment. The molecular mechanism of action at the organelle level is less clear, although mitochondrial protein synthesis is clearly impaired at high levels of mutant mtDNA, and the synthesis of at least one abnormal polypeptide has been reported (Dunbar et al., 1996). Indeed, a mutation that results in a functional deficit of any tRNA may be predicted to have similar effects. The np 7445 mutation, for example, impairs the accumulation of tRNA-ser(UCN) (Reid et al., 1997), acting presumably at the level of RNA processing, since the mutation falls one base pair beyond the tRNA 3' end. A long-favoured model for how heteroplasmic deletions may impair mitochondrial function is via distortion of the ratios of different tRNAs inside mitochondria, causing a deficit of one or more species (Hayashi et al., 1991). An alternative model to account for the pathological effects of rearranged mtDNAs, both deletions and partial duplications, is that an abnormal fusion peptide is potentially encoded across rearrangement break-points, due to the joining of part of a *bona fide* protein-coding sequence to sequences from a completely different gene. The accumulation of such a fusion peptide has been clearly demonstrated in at least one case (Hayashi et al., 1991), but has not been systematically investigated by sensitive methods, so therefore the question of whether such products are present generally remains unresolved.

Nuclear genes involved in mitochondrial protein quality control

The inference that a variety of different mtDNA mutations which promote the synthesis of abnormal translation products are associated with the phenotype of SNHI leads to an important and obvious prediction, namely that any nuclear gene which can mutate with a similar 'molecular' effect is also a candidate gene in SNHI. The mitochondrial translation system depends on over 100 nuclear-coded gene products, including about 80 ribosomal proteins distinct from those of the cytosolic ribosome (Pietromonaco et al., 1991), 20 aminoacyl-tRNA synthetases, also, based on the precedent of yeast, largely distinct from their cytosolic counterparts (Tzagoloff et al., 1986), plus a largely uncharacterized set of gene products involved in maturation of mitochondrial tRNA.

Particularly strong candidates for nuclear genetic involvement in SNHI via this route are those genes whose products are known to interact with the critical regions of mtDNA-encoded RNAs in which SNHI-associated mutations have been identified. The best example is that of the genes encoding the protein components of the ribosomal accuracy centre. At least three such proteins have been identified in bacteria, based on mutations which suppress or are suppressed by rRNA mutations in the accuracy domain, thus modifying susceptibility to aminoglycosides (Alksne et al., 1993). These are the ribosomal proteins designated S12, S4 and S5 in *E. coli*. Mutations in the bacterial genes for these proteins also compensate for one another, as do mutations in the gene (tufA) for elongation factor EF-Tu (Kraal et al., 1995).

The genetic data in bacteria strongly suggest not only that the human homologues of these genes are candidates for causing SNHI, but, moreover, that the phenotypic 'outcome' in humans is likely to depend on interactions between mitochondrial genotype, nuclear genotype and environmental factors.

A scheme outlining this in relation to the ribosomal accuracy centre is shown in Figure 20.1. The 'wild-type' human mitochondrial ribosome is regarded as insensitive to aminoglycosides, but the np 1555 mutation alters the structure of the mitoribosomal accuracy centre such that in combination with aminoglycosides a level of translational impairment results that causes a defect in cells of the auditory system. A similar effect might be predicted to occur from mutations in the genes for the mitoribosomal homologues of the *E. coli* S12, S4 or S5 genes, or even *tufA*. Thus, aminoglycoside ototoxicity may be predicted to occur in individuals without the np 1555 or any other predisposing mtDNA mutation, but who have susceptibility mutations in nuclear genes for the mitoribosomal accuracy centre. These would theoretically show Mendelian inheritance, but given the requirement for an environmental interaction, plus the possibility that the phenotype might manifest only in a homozygote, occurrence would more likely appear to be sporadic.

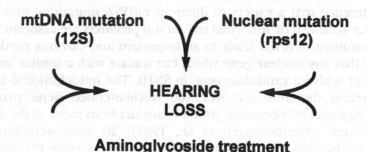

mtDNA mutation (12S)   Nuclear mutation (rps12)

HEARING LOSS

Aminoglycoside treatment

Figure 20.1 Possible interactions between nuclear and mitochondrial genotype, plus aminoglycosides, in sensorineural hearing impairment consequent on defects in translational accuracy in mitochondria.

We have screened a group of 17 unrelated individuals from China with aminoglycoside ototoxicity for the np 1555 mutation, and found it in only one case (apart from the monozygotic twin brother of the individual concerned). Although we cannot rule out the possibility of a different mtDNA mutation in the remaining 16, a more likely explanation is that susceptibility in these individuals is due to a nuclear gene defect, and we are currently examining this hypothesis in relation to the gene for human mitoribosomal protein S12, described in more detail below.

A further prediction is that some individuals might develop aminoglycoside-independent SNHI as a result of a defect in the mitoribosomal accuracy centre, if nuclear and mitochondrial mutations that individually require aminoglycoside interaction to affect phenotype are brought together in the same person. Thus, the np 1555 mutation may be silent in a wild-type nuclear background, unless the individual is treated with the drug, but may cause translational inaccuracy and hence SNHI in a mutant nuclear background where one of the interacting ribosomal protein genes is also altered. This would explain neatly why some np 1555-positive families, especially those of Mediterranean origin, contain individuals who develop deafness without aminoglycoside treatment. Once again, we would predict a correlation between phenotype and genotype for mitoribosomal protein S12 or other genes for the accuracy centre, which is also easily testable.

In addition to effects at the level of the translation system *per se*, the hypothesis that some cell-type(s) of the auditory system are hypersensitive to the presence of abnormal mitochondrial translation products raises the possibility that genes involved normally in the turnover of such molecules should also be considered as candidate genes in SNHI. A number of such genes have been characterized in yeast (Rep et al., 1995), and a similar role in mammalian mitochondria is implied by the discovery of clear mammalian homologues of them. Two candidates particularly worthy of consideration are the related ATPase/proteases of the AAA family designated AFG3 and RCA1. These genes encode proteins that appear to have a dual function inside mitochondria. On the one hand, they act as chaperones or assembly factors in the delivery of mtDNA-encoded polypeptides to the multisubunit complexes in the mitochondrial inner membrane of which they form part. On the other, they function in the turnover of such polypeptides if misfolded, mistranslated, oxidatively damaged or for some other reason not incorporated into the appropriate enzyme complex. In yeast, the two members of the gene family perform this role for distinct sets of mtDNA-encoded polypeptides, although there is a small amount of overlap in their substrate specificity.

Why hearing impairment should result from such a mechanism remains mysterious. However, an obvious explanation would be that a key component of the mitochondrial protein quality control system is simply limiting in the target cell-type, e.g. hair cells, such that its ability to tolerate defects in mitochondrial protein synthesis is much lower than that of other cell-types. This may be because a critical gene, e.g. a human homologue of the AFG3/RCA1 family, is expressed at only low levels in this cell-type, or alternatively because a critical component of the apparatus of mitochondrial protein synthesis/metabolism is encoded by a multi-gene family expressed in a tissue-specific fashion, and that the isologue expressed in the auditory system is functionally less adapted than those expressed elsewhere.

Strategy for identifying nuclear genes involved in 'mitochondrial deafness'

Working from the foregoing hypothesis, we are attempting to isolate and characterize some of the key genes referred to above, both from human and mouse, in order to address the issues raised. In each case we aim to answer four questions:

* Is the gene linked to an SNHI phenotype in humans (or in a mouse model)?
* Does the expression pattern of the gene indicate it as a likely candidate for the limiting factor causing susceptibility of the auditory system to mitochondrial dysfunction?
* Can we manipulate expression of the gene so as to create a cellular (or eventually perhaps a whole organism) model for 'mitochondrial deafness', in which we can study the pathogenic process?
* Can we manipulate expression of the gene so as to complement and thus correct the effects of SNHI-associated mutations in mtDNA, thus opening a potential route to gene therapy?

Our strategy is made much easier by the rapid advance of genetic knowledge, based on the one hand on the recent completion of the DNA sequence of a model eukaryote, the yeast *Saccharomyces cerevisiae*, in which it is particularly simple to evaluate mitochondrial phenotypes, and on the other, the explosion of data on human and mouse expressed genes, via the expressed sequence tag (EST) projects. Combined with cDNA cloning via redundant PCR, this has enabled us to isolate probably full-length cDNA homologues of the human genes for mitochondrial leucyl-tRNA synthetase and mitoribosomal protein S12, as well as a partial cDNA for a human member of the AFG3/RCA1 gene family. We have also progressed, collaboratively, on the characterization of human nuclear genes for mitochondrial EF-Tu.

Our strategy is outlined in Figure 20.2. In many ways it is the exact opposite of the positional cloning approach taken elsewhere. Instead of mapping a disease gene, then cloning it from positional data and resources, we start from the gene of interest, then map it. To make sense of the data obtained, we rely upon the disease gene mapping work underway elsewhere. Because the number of SNHI-associated genes probably exceeds 50, fewer than half of which have been thus far mapped, we will in many cases not know for some time if a gene we are able to characterize and map is or is not involved in the phenotype. When a co-localization is revealed, however, we can proceed rapidly to mutational analysis, to confirm or refute the hypothesis of involvement.

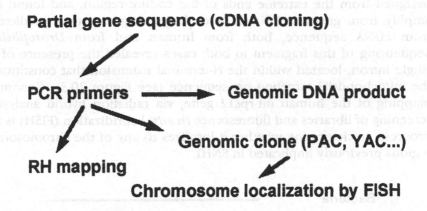

Partial gene sequence (cDNA cloning)

PCR primers ⟶ **Genomic DNA product**

Genomic clone (PAC, YAC...)

RH mapping

Chromosome localization by FISH

Figure 20.2 The candidate gene approach to disease gene identification. RH-radiation hybrid. FISH-fluorescence in situ hybridization. PAC-P1 artificial chromosome. YAC-Yeast artificial chromosome.

Metazoan genes for mitoribosomal protein S12

The mitochondrial homologue of *E. coli* ribosomal protein S12 is encoded by a mitochondrial gene in plants and some protozoa, but by a nuclear gene in fungi and metazoans. Alignment of sequences of ribosomal protein S12 from bacteria, chloroplasts and mitochondria (Figure 20.3) shows clearly that this is a distinct and well conserved gene family. The nuclear gene that encodes the cytosolic counterpart of this protein is only very distantly related by sequence, allowing unambiguous identification of the gene that encodes the mitochondrial isologue in any newly studied eukaryote. The gene shows some highly conserved regions. Analysis of mutants in *E. coli* and other eubacteria that confer altered aminoglycoside sensitivity has identified two specific regions of the protein that are critical for its function in mediating translational fidelity and the interaction of the ribosome with aminoglycoside antibiotics (Timms et al., 1992).

The gene has also been previously characterized in the fruit fly *Drosophila* (Royden et al., 1987), because mutations in it result in an interesting behavioural phenotype of potential relevance to human SNHI. The gene, designated *tko* (*technical knock-out*) because of the associated phenotype of stress-induced paralysis, encodes a polypeptide highly homologous to the one studied in bacteria, chloroplasts and plant mitochondria, but with an N-terminal extension characteristic of mitochondrially targeted proteins.

Analysis of EST data has allowed the identification of sets of overlapping cDNAs encoding the human and mouse homologues. The sequence of the entire coding region of the gene from these two species was derived by us from representative cDNA clones. PCR primers were designed from the extreme ends of the coding region, and found to amplify, from genomic DNA, a much larger fragment than predicted from cDNA sequence, both from human and from *Drosophila*. Sequencing of this fragment in both cases revealed the presence of a single intron, located within the N-terminal extension that constitutes the mitochondrial targeting pre-sequence (see Figure 20.3). Genomic mapping of the human mt-rps12 gene, via radiation hybrid analysis, screening of libraries and fluorescence *in situ* hybridization (FISH) is in progress, to determine whether it localizes to any of the chromosome regions previously implicated in SNHI.

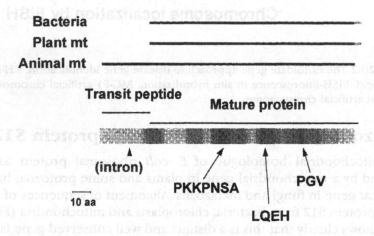

Figure 20.3 Schematic representation of ribosomal protein S12 sequences inferred from DNA sequence data. Shading indicates degree of phylogenetic conservation of the amino acid sequence, comparing sequences from bacteria, and mitochondria of four widely separated taxonomic groups (sunflower, *Drosophila*, human and mouse). Darkest shading indicates highest conservation, computed as a moving average of identity across five adjacent residues. Invariant runs of amino acid sequence are indicated by use of the standard one-letter code (Strachan & Read, 1996).

Interestingly, all of the mitochondrial rps12 sequences analysed show a substitution with respect to the bacterial gene at the residue designated K87 in the *E. coli* gene (Figure 20.4). This residue is implicated in translational fidelity. Substitution of glutamine or arginine at this position in bacteria results in aminoglycoside resistance, in other words a hyper-faithful ribosome. All of the mitochondrial S12 genes appear to have Q (glutamine) at this position except for *Paramecium* which has arginine. The strong implication is that the mitochondrial ribosome is naturally aminoglycoside-resistant, which accords with the known fact that eukaryotic cells are not affected by this class of drugs. Arguably the decreased rate of translation which is associated with this change can be tolerated in mitochondria, where the 'per gene' rate of protein synthesis is much lower than for nuclear genes coding for subunits of the same enzyme complexes. A back-mutation at this position, or a mutation at a nearby residue, may well confer drug sensitivity on the mitochondrial ribosome and may thus be predicted as a candidate mutation in human 'mitochondrial' SNHI.

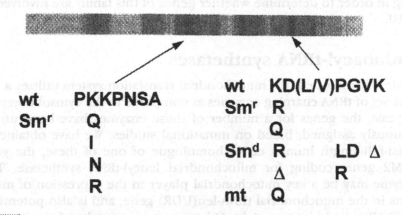

Figure 20.4 Schematic representation of ribosomal protein S12 sequences of bacteria and mitochondria, as in Figure 20.3. Bacterial mutations conferring streptomycin resistance (Sm^r) or dependence (Sm^d) and the mitochondrial sequence found in all metazoans, are indicated by use of the standard one-letter amino acid code. Deletion of an amino acid residue is indicated by Δ.

We have also analysed the mutant allele in the *Drosophila tko* mutant. This exhibits a novel substitution (L56H), located close to the major conserved motif within which lies another residue implicated in translational fidelity and aminoglycoside susceptibility in bacteria. No other substitutions with respect to the wild-type gene are evident, and we are verifying that the mutant allele is expressed at the same level as wild-type. Perhaps most intriguingly, the physiological effect of this mutation in the fly appears to be at the level of mechanosensory transduction (Engel et al., 1994). This provides a close parallel with human mitochondrial SNHI. It leaves, or rather emphasizes, the mystery as to why an impairment of mitochondrial translation should specifically affect mechanosensor cells.

Mammalian genes for members of the AFG3/RCA1 gene family

EST analysis has also revealed mouse and human expressed sequences corresponding to at least one member of the AFG3/RCA1 gene family, which we refer to here arbitrarily as AFG3. Once again, we have been able to design PCR primers that amplify a segment of the gene, containing an intron, from genomic DNA. We have used these primers to isolate a genomic clone from a PAC library (supplied by HGMP Resource Centre, Cambridge), which contains the gene defined by these primers. Gene localization by radiation hybrid mapping and FISH is in progress. Based on EST analysis the *AFG3/RCA1* gene family comprizes at least two members in humans, at least three in the mouse and probably more. Additional candidates will therefore need to be evaluated by mapping in order to determine whether genes of this family are involved in SNHI.

Aminoacyl-tRNA synthetases

As already indicated, the mitochondrial translation system utilizes a distinct set of tRNA charging enzymes as compared to the cytosolic system. In yeast, the genes for a number of these enzymes have been unambiguously assigned, based on mutational studies. We have obtained a quasi-full-length human cDNA homologue of one of these, the yeast NAM2 gene, coding for mitochondrial leucyl-tRNA synthetase. This enzyme may be a key mitochondrial player in the expression of mutations in the mitochondrial tRNA-leu(UUR) gene, and is also potentially an SNHI gene in its own right. Other yeast genes coding for mitochondrial aminoacyl-tRNA synthetases may be tentatively inferred from sequence, as they are, in general, much more similar to eubacterial homologues than to those of the cytosolic translational apparatus. One such case is that of the mitochondrial seryl-tRNA synthetase. Although this has not yet been identified genetically, sequence data imply that it almost certainly corresponds to the yeast open reading frame YHR011w, which has informed our search for the human homologue.

Next steps

Judging the likely importance of different genetic contributors to a heterogenous disorder is extremely hazardous in the absence of a substantial body of data. Genes thus far implicated in SNHI, either via human mutations or implied from animal models, include several distinct classes, notably genes for cytoskeletal components, ion channels, transcription factors and components of the mitochondrial translation system. Some of these discoveries can be fitted into a simple conceptual framework, whereas others, notably the discovery of mitochondrial involvement, neither conformed to pre-existing paradigms, nor can be built easily into an all-embracing model.

The relative importance, at the population level, of different contributory mutations may not reflect the relative significance of the various genes to processes at the cellular or physiological level. For example, Duchenne muscular dystrophy involves a gene that codes for what would otherwise have been regarded as a minor component of the acto-myosin complex. The importance of dystrophin as a genetic target in the disease has much more to do with the unusual structure of the gene, making it vulnerable to mutations that disrupt its integrity. Other factors influencing the importance of a given gene in disease include the tissue-selectivity of its expression pattern, and questions of genetic redundancy. Even a relatively 'minor' gene for a common metabolic function can be a target in tissue-specific disease, if its expression pattern is highly tissue-restricted, e.g. if it is a member of a multi-gene family.

The approach we are taking to identify genes involved in SNHI makes no presumptions about the likely prevalence of 'mitochondrial' as opposed to 'non-mitochondrial' causes of the disorder, but simply takes as its starting point the premise that mitochondrial protein quality control is important for the proper functioning of the auditory system. Dissecting the genetic factors that govern this will help us towards a better understanding of the system, and towards the possibility of eventual therapeutic intervention.

Conclusions

Many different mutations in mitochondrial DNA are associated with both syndromal and non-syndromal forms of SNHI. A unifying hypothesis is that all of these result in the accumulation of mistranslated polypeptides, either by impairing translational fidelity, or by causing tRNA insufficiency. Mitochondrial protein synthesis depends on more than 100 nuclear-coded gene products, many of which have predictable roles in tRNA function and translational fidelity. This leads to the prediction of an important new class of nuclear candidate genes in hearing impairment. We are working to clone and characterize a number of such genes, to map them in the human genome, and to create variants for expression in mammalian cells to measure their effects on mitochondrial protein synthesis, respiratory metabolism and cell survival, and interactions with mutant mtDNAs. Current efforts are focusing on the genes for mitochondrial leucyl- and seryl-tRNA synthetases, mitoribosomal protein S12, and a mammalian homologue of the yeast AFG3 gene, which is required for the turnover of mistranslated proteins inside mitochondria.

Acknowledgements

Our work is supported by the Finnish Academy, the EU Human Capital and Mobility and Biomed 2 Programmes and the Juselius Foundation.

Chapter 21
A mitochondrial point mutation at position 7472 causes early onset hearing impairment and late onset neurological symptoms. Report of a Dutch family and a comparison with a Sicilian family

RJH ENSINK, PLM HUYGEN, HAM MARRES, K VERHOEVEN,
G VAN CAMP, CWRJ CREMERS and GW PADBERG

Introduction

Many previously unclassified neurological syndromes have been linked to mitochondrial mutations over the past few years (DiMauro et al., 1985). Largely because of its small size (16 659 base pairs), the mitochondrial DNA has emerged as among the best studied DNA in humans. In general, the most common mutations are deletions, duplications and point mutations (Lestienne, 1994). Large scale rearrangements give a clinical picture compatible with ocular myopathy; most common is the Kearns–Sayre syndrome with or without chronic progressive external ophthalmoplegia (CPEO). Several distinct syndromes, usually with maternal inheritance, are caused by point mutations, including LHON, MERRF and MELAS syndromes (DiMauro et al., 1985). Many maternally inherited syndromes show overlapping clinical symptoms, even with different mutations. In approximately 70% of these maternally inherited syndromes hearing impairment is an associated finding (Gold et al., 1994).

Two mitochondrial mutations have been associated with hearing impairment as the only symptom of disease. The first detected mutation, a A1555G substitution in the *12S rRNA* gene, is associated with aminoglycoside-induced deafness (Prezant et al., 1993). The second, a C7445G substitution in the tRNASer(UCN)gene, has been detected in two unrelated families originating from Scotland and New Zealand (Fischel Ghodsian et al., 1995).

A third, large Dutch family was found with a maternal trait of hearing impairment with full penetrance and additional, mainly late onset, neurological signs and symptoms in the proband only. The family carries an insertion of a C nucleotide at position 7442 of the mitochondrial genome. This mutation was previously described in a family originating from Sicily (Tiranti et al., 1995). We describe and compare the families and their probands.

Dutch and Sicilian families with 7472 INSC mutation — a comparison

Dutch family

The pedigree of the Dutch family consists of 69 maternally related family members (Figure 21.1). High-frequency hearing impairment was the only presenting symptom in 29 of 32 (91%) family members. In the index case, and most affected members, hearing deteriorated from the age of approximately 20 years, although some relatives reported an age of onset of 45 years. Tinnitus and vertigo, which gradually became worse, were present in the proband from the age of 18 years. Many family members have developed similar complaints. Vestibular dysfunction was demonstrated in the majority of hearing impaired family members (13/20).

One brother died from a previously unclassified progressive disease believed to be some type of amyotrophic lateral sclerosis which started at the age of 40 years. In another brother, focal myoclonus was reported. No other family members exhibited neurological complaints. The proband exhibited similar neurological complaints consisting of dysarthria, truncal ataxia and distal polyneuropathy from the age of 30 years. No focal myoclonus was observed. To evaluate neuromuscular complaints, muscle biopsy was performed which revealed numerous altered mitochondria with paracrystalline inclusions and lipid accumulation. The superior cerebellar vermis appeared atrophic on magnetic resonance imaging (MRI) scan (Figure 21.2).

Sicilian family

The pedigree of the previously reported Sicilian family consists of 20 maternally related members (Tiranti et al., 1995). Only in three individuals was hearing impairment, the sole manifestation of the mutation. Although not specified, hearing impairment was the presenting symptom in the majority of the neurologically affected individuals. Hearing impairment generally started at a young age, ranging between 15–28

years, and was often accompanied by tinnitus and 'episodes of vertigo'.
No data on vestibular function were available.

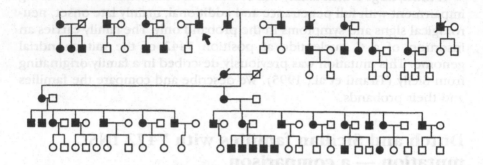

Figure 21.1 Pedigree of the Dutch family. Arrow points at the proband.

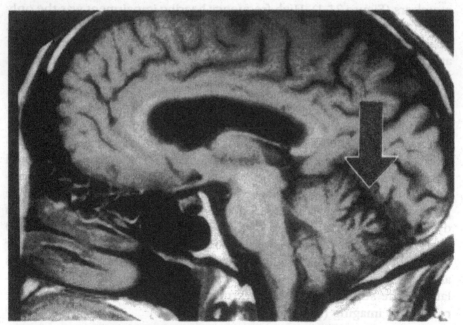

Figure 21.2 Characteristic abnormalities found in the Dutch proband also
described in the Sicilian proband. Arrow points at atrophy of the cerebellar vermis
on MRI.

Neurological complaints were more marked and presented earlier.
Characteristic complaints were focal myoclonus, dysarthria, gait ataxia
and mild generalized hypotonia with dysaesthesia. A niece of the proband
suffered, at the age of 25, from a neurological syndrome characterized by
optic neuritis, ataxia and diplopia and moderate mental deterioration

without tinnitus, hearing impairment or vertigo. The proband presented with focal myoclonic jerks of the abdominal muscles at the age of 28; over the previous three years he had experienced hearing impairment and tinnitus. Auditory brainstem responses (ABR) disclosed cochlear and retro-cochlear characteristics. Muscle biopsy showed mitochondria with altered cristae and para-crystalline inclusions. Atrophy of the superior cerebellar vermis was found on computer tomography (CT) and MRI examination. Table 21.1 compares both probands and their families.

Table 21.1 Comparison of the Dutch and Sicilian probands

	Dutch proband	*Sicilian proband*
Age at examination (years)	68	35
Hearing impairment (onset age)	+ (18 years)	+ (25 years)
Average hearing loss	68 dB (high Fletcher index)	45 dB
Tinnitus	+	+
Focal myoclonic jerks	Absent	+
Ataxic gait	+	+
Dysarthria	+	+
Truncal ataxia	+	Absent
Dysaethesia lower limbs	+	+
Eyes — optic fundi	Normal	Normal
Eyes — cataract	Present	Not examined
ECG	Unexplained cardiac conduction deficit	Normal
Renal function	High levels of urea, creatinine	Not investigated
Muscle biopsy	altered large mitochondria; abundant intramuscular fat accumulation	altered large mitochondria with concentric cristae
Red-ragged fibres	Absent	Absent
Maternal great-grandmother	No consanguinity	Consanguineous marriage
Hearing impairment	Starting at high frequencies	Starting at high frequencies
Hearing impairment in family	Initial and only manifestation	Initial manifestation
Neurological symptoms in family	Infrequent	More prominent (early onset)

Discussion

Many similarities were found comparing these two families which have the same mutation in the mitochondrial tRNAser(UCN) gene — insertion of an extra C at position 7472. In particular both probands showed a remarkably similar clinical picture. Their families differ especially in the degree of hearing impairment and the age of onset of neurological symptoms.

The observation of maternally inherited hearing impairment may trigger detection of a mitochondrial mutation in a family where the proband presents with an unclear and undefined neurological syndrome. It may be that the prevalence of mitochondrial hearing impairment is higher than recognized at present. Further research will show whether genuine non-syndromal types of mitochondrial hearing impairment exist or, as might be expected, oligosymptomatic types with hearing impairment as the most prominent and/or the earliest abnormality, occur more frequently.

Chapter 22
Genetic study of mitochondrially inherited sensorineural hearing impairment in eight large families from Spain and Cuba

M SARDUY, I DEL CASTILLO, M VILLAMAR, L ROMERO,
C HERRAIZ, FJ HERNANDEZ, MC TAPIA, C MAGARIÑO,
D MÉNDEZ DEL CASTILLO, I MENÉNDEZ-ALEJO,
R RAMIREZ-CAMACHO, B ARELLANO, C MORALES, J BELLON
and F MORENO

Introduction

Maternally inherited non-syndromal hearing impairment (NSHI) can be caused by point mutations in the mitochondrial genome. Up to now, two independent mutations have been characterized: the A1555G mutation in the mitochondrial 12S rRNA gene (Prezant et al., 1993), and the T7445C mutation in the mitochondrial gene for the tRNASer(UCN) (Reid et al., 1994). The A1555G mutation is usually related to ototoxicity from treatment with aminoglycoside antibiotics, and it has been inferred that this mutation confers susceptibility to the ototoxic effects of these drugs (Hutchin et al., 1993; Prezant et al., 1993). However, the A1555G mutation has also been reported in an Arab-Israeli pedigree in the absence of treatment by these drugs (Jaber et al., 1992; Prezant et al., 1993). The T7445C mutation is also responsible for NSHI and seems to be unrelated to drug-induced ototoxicity (Reid et al., 1994).

In this work, eight large families were analysed, five from Spain and three from Cuba, affected by NSHI with a suspected maternal inheritance pattern. The clinical features of hearing impairment in each family were studied, and a search for mitochondrial mutations was undertaken.

121

Materials and methods

Family data

Clinical examination was performed on all patients and their living maternal relatives who were available for the study. By use of pure tone audiometry (PTA), the frequencies tested by air conduction were 250, 500, 1000, 2000, 4000 and 8000 Hz, and the frequencies tested by bone conduction were 250, 500, 1000, 2000 and 4000 Hz. Otoscopic examination, tympanometry with acoustic reflex testing, and tuning fork tests were carried out systematically to rule out a conductive hearing loss. For all patients, there was no evidence of environmental factors such as exposure to noise, otoacoustic trauma or ear infections. Ototoxicity due to aminoglycoside antibiotics was investigated from the clinical histories and by interviewing the patients. No syndromal features were revealed on examination of the eyes, skin or renal function.

Mutation detection

DNA was extracted from peripheral blood by the salting out method (Miller et al., 1988). PCR amplification of a 342 bp DNA product including the mutation site was performed in a total volume of 50 μl in a Perkin–Elmer 9600 DNA amplifier, using standard conditions and previously published primers (Shoffner et al., 1995). The amplification programme consisted of an initial denaturation step at 94°C for 2 min, followed by 30 cycles of denaturation at 94°C for 40 sec, annealing at 50°C for 45 sec, and extension at 72°C for 30 sec. Digestion of the 342 bp PCR product with *Alw26I* was performed according to the recommendations of the enzyme manufacturer, and the digestion products were resolved on 2% agarose gels containing 0.5 μg/μl ethidium bromide.

DNA sequencing was carried out by the dideoxynucleotide chain-termination method, using T7 Sequenase, version 2.0 (USB–Amersham).

Results and discussion

All the pedigrees included in this study were detected during routine collection of families affected by sensorineural hearing impairment, a search that was performed with the aim of mapping novel NSHI genes by linkage analysis. A superficial look at the patterns of inheritance of the hearing impairment in these eight pedigrees (Figure 22.1) would classify them as Mendelian (X-linked in families S004 and S027, and autosomal dominant with incomplete penetrance in the other six families). However, more careful observation reveals that deafness is maternally inherited in all cases. Since no other clinical sign was associated with hearing impairment in any of the families, we began searching for those point mutations in the mitochondrial genome that have been reported to cause NSHI.

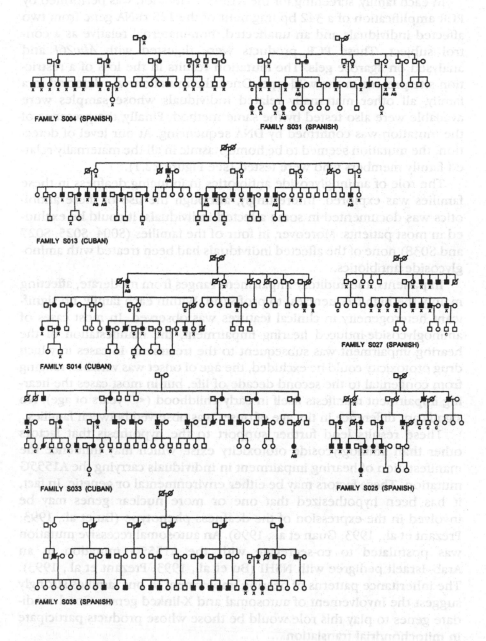

Figure 22.1 Families affected by maternally inherited NSHI which were included in the study. Solid symbols: severe to profound hearing impairment. Half-shaded symbols: moderate hearing impairment. Letters below the symbols: X, individual whose sample was available and who carries the A1555G mutation in homoplasmic form; C, control individual who does not carry the A1555G mutation; AG, individual treated with one or more aminoglycoside antibiotics.

In each family, screening for the A1555G mutation was performed by PCR amplification of a 342 bp fragment of the 12S rRNA gene from two affected individuals and an unaffected, non-maternal relative as a control subject. These PCR products were digested with *Alw26I* and analysed on agarose gels. The mutation results in the loss of a restriction site present in the wild-type. Once the mutation was detected in a family, all other maternally related individuals whose samples were available were also tested by the same method. Finally, the presence of the mutation was confirmed by DNA sequencing. At our level of detection, the mutation seemed to be homoplasmic in all the maternally related family members who were tested (see Figure 22.1).

The role of aminoglycoside antibiotics in inducing deafness in these families was explored. Interestingly, although the use of these antibiotics was documented in some affected individuals, it could be excluded in most patients. Moreover, in four of the families (S004, S025, S027 and S038) none of the affected individuals had been treated with aminoglycoside antibiotics.

In patients, the auditory impairment ranges from moderate, affecting mainly the high frequencies, to profound. Within each family, no significant heterogeneity in clinical features was observed. In most cases of aminoglycoside-induced hearing impairment, the manifestation of the hearing impairment was subsequent to the treatment. In cases in which drug ototoxicity could be excluded, the age of onset was variable, ranging from congenital to the second decade of life, but in most cases the hearing impairment manifests itself in early childhood (<7 years of age). No significant difference in the age of onset was observed between families.

These results lend further support to the hypothesis that factors other than aminoglycoside ototoxicity exist, which may influence the manifestation of hearing impairment in individuals carrying the A1555G mutation. These factors may be either environmental or genetic. In fact, it has been hypothesized that one or more nuclear genes may be involved in the expression of the deafness phenotype (Bu et al., 1993; Prezant et al., 1993; Guan et al., 1996). An autosomal recessive mutation was postulated to co-segregate with the A1555G mutation in an Arab–Israeli pedigree with NSHI (Bu et al., 1993; Prezant et al., 1993). The inheritance patterns of hearing impairment in our families strongly suggest the involvement of autosomal and X-linked genes. Good candidate genes to play this role would be those whose products participate in mitochondrial translation.

The eight pedigrees reported here represent 16% of our series of families affected by NSHI which were collected for genetic linkage studies. Although our sample may be biased due to the need to collect families with more than five affected individuals, our data suggest that the prevalence of mitochondrially inherited hearing impairment may be much higher than currently expected.

Conclusions

NSHI due to the A1555G mutation in the mitochondrial 12S rRNA gene is usually related to sensitivity to aminoglycoside antibiotics. Nevertheless, it has also been reported in an Arab–Israeli pedigree in the absence of such treatment. Eight large families were studied, five from Spain and three from Cuba, affected by NSHI with a suspected maternal inheritance pattern. The A1555G mutation was detected in homoplasmic form in all of the maternally related members who were tested in each family. In our set of patients, the auditory impairment ranges from moderate, affecting mainly the high frequencies, to profound. The age of onset is variable, ranging from congenital to the second decade of life. Interestingly, although use of aminoglycoside antibiotics was documented in some affected individuals, it could be excluded in many other patients. These results give further support to the hypothesis that additional factors, either genetic or environmental, exist which may influence the manifestation of deafness in individuals carrying the A1555G mutation. These data also suggest that the prevalence of mitochondrially inherited hearing impairment may be much higher than currently assumed.

Acknowledgements

We thank the members of the families included in this study for their kind cooperation, T Carril and A Cardeñosa for collecting the blood samples, Professor F Olaizola for his enthusiastic support, and J Sainz for critical reading of the manuscript. This work was supported by grants from the European Community (PL 951324) and the Fondo de Investigaciones Sanitarias de la Seguridad Social (no. 96/1556) (Ministerio de Sanidad y Consumo, Spain).

Chapter 23
Hearing impairment in patients with a mitochondrial point mutation

E ORZAN, L BARTOLOMEI, V MAGNAVITA and E ARSLAN

Introduction

At present, the clinical identification of mitochondrial mutations with aetiological roles in hearing impairment (and other disorders) can be challenging, because many known mitochondrial diseases show only partial penetrance and considerable symptomatic variability. Family history, if characterized by maternal transmission, can provide a good diagnostic clue. Mitochondrial origin should also be considered where hearing impairment is part of a multisystem condition particularly affecting tissues with high metabolic activity, such as muscle or brain (Reardon et al., 1995).

Hearing impairment is a common finding in syndromal neuromuscular mitochondrial pathology. In mitochondrial encephalopathy with lactic acidosis and stroke-like episodes (MELAS), hearing impairment is described as a part of the symptom cluster characterized by stroke-like episodes, lactic acidosis, red-ragged fibres on the muscle biopsy and possible additional symptoms, such as mental retardation, focal or generalized seizures, recurrent headache and vomiting and short stature (Cianfaloni et al., 1992). However, other cases of MELAS show only partial expression of the syndrome with great symptom variability (Moraes et al., 1993). In addition, other phenotypes have been described in association with the point mutation affecting this mitochondrial gene (Martinuzzi et al., 1992). There are descriptions of several families with mitochondrial mutation in whom sensorineural hearing impairment and diabetes mellitus occur with significant penetrance and not always together, without other neurological symptoms (Ballinger et al., 1992; Van den Ouweland et al., 1992; Remes et al., 1993, Kadowaki et al., 1994).

This paper describes the audiological findings and the longitudinal

126

description of audiometric features in three hearing impaired women with an identical point mutation which affects the mtDNA gene coding for tRNA Leu(UUR) at the nucleotide 3243. The clinical phenotype of the three patients does not correspond to the MELAS syndrome.

Families

One patient presented with myocardiopathy and ocular myopathy. The second had intellectual decline and myoclonus, and only diabetes was present in the third. Moreover, the probands' relatives carrying the mutation show a great variability in phenotypic expression together with a frequent presence of hearing impairment. Family A is described in Table 23.1 and the family tree is shown in Figure 23.1. The auditory brainstem responses (ABRs) for the proband of this family at the time of onset of hearing impairment are shown in Table 23.2.

Pure tone audiometry, stapedial reflex measurements, ABR and DPOAE were also performed in subjects II-2, II-4 and III-6 with normal results.

Table 23.1 Family A

Case	Age (years)	Sex	Clinical picture	Mutated mtDNA (%)	
				Muscle	Blood
I-1	68	F	Asymptomatic	55	<2
II-1	45	M	Asymptomatic	53	30
II-2	43	F	Asymptomatic	78	40
II-4	41	F	Asymptomatic	72	28
II-5	29	F	Asymptomatic	74	52
III-4	21	M	Short, profound hearing loss, seizures, dementia, MELAS, deceased due to myocardiopathy	94	75
III-5	20	F	**Myoclonus, hearing loss, intellectual decline**	85	59

The hearing deficit, longitudinally studied in the three probands, appears to be of predominantly cochlear origin, although a retro-cochlear involvement could not be excluded in the diabetic patient. Audiometric patterns were variable and progression was unpredictable. It is not clear if the progression of hearing loss can be a marker for a more severe course of the disease.

Considering all the members of the three families carrying the mtDNA mutation (25 subjects), hearing impairment was reported as always present (nine subjects) with other symptoms of mitochondrial disorders (short stature, myocardiopathy, encephalomyopathy, mental retardation, seizures, diabetes mellitus). Pure tone audiometry, stapedial reflex measurement, ABR and distortion product otoacoustic

Table 23.2 ABR of the proband of Family A

Right ear*

Wave	Latency (ms)	Normal values (95%)	Probability of wave identification (%)
I	1.87	1.4–2.0	100
III	3.66	3.4–4.3	100
V	5.53	5.1–6.1	100
I–III	1.79	1.8–2.5	
III–V	1.87	1.2–2.1	
I–V	3.66	3.5–4.3	

ΔV −0.072 (Ref. 25 dB HL: −0.6:0.5)

Left ear**

Wave	Latency (ms)	Normal values (95%)	Probability of wave identification (%)
I	1.89	1.6–2.2	87
III	3.77	3.6–4.6	100
V	5.66	5.3–6.4	100
I–III	1.88	1.8–2.5	
III–V	1.89	1.3–2.2	
I–V	3.77	3.5–4.3	

*Pure tone threshold average 2–4 kHz: 25 dB HL, reference data calculated for 65 dB SL.

**Pure tone threshold average 2–4 kHz: 35 dB HL, reference data calculated for 55 dB SL.

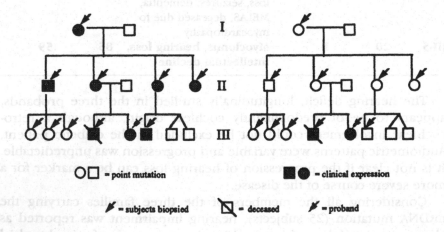

Figure 23.1 Family tree of one patient with progressive sensorineural hearing loss of cochlear origin. Table 23.1 shows the clinical expression and the percentages of mutated mtDNA in muscle and blood of biopsied subjects (the proband is given in bold characters).

emissions (DPOAE) were performed on four asymptomatic subjects carrying the mutation and showed normal results.

Only a minority of subjects with described point mutation show symptoms of mitochondrial pathology.

Although hearing impairment is a common finding in patients with mitochondrial mutations and there is increasing published evidence of a mitochondrial aetiology in progressive hearing losses without associated symptoms. Patient management and parental counselling are particularly challenging in terms of the symptomatic variability of the disease and the unpredictable progression of the hearing impairment.

Chapter 24
Prevalence of the base pair 3243 mutation of the *tRNALeu* gene in the mitochondrial DNA in a population-based cohort of patients with sensorineural hearing impairment

S UIMONEN, I HASSINEN, M SORRI and K MAJAMAA

Abstract

Sensorineural hearing impairment (SNHI) is a frequent manifestation of the mitochondrial syndrome (MELAS) mitochondrial encephalopathy, lactic acidosis, stroke-like episodes. The most common molecular defect in this syndrome is a point mutation at base pair (bp) 3243 in the gene encoding the transfer RNA for leucine. In addition to being associated with the specific syndrome MELAS, SNHI can also be expressed as a non-syndromal symptom. Point mutations at bp 1555 and 7445 have been observed in such cases. Furthermore, it has been shown that the point mutation at bp 1555 is a predisposing factor for aminoglycoside induced cochlear damage.

No data exist on the frequency of these mutations among genetic SNHI.

A population-based sampling of patients with SNHI was carried out. The register of patients supplied with hearing aids included 6840 patients. By use of defined clinical criteria (age, type of hearing impairment, non-acquired hearing impairment) a cohort of 242 patients was identified; the cohort was studied for family history by use of a questionnaire.

Sixty-five cases (probands) with an apparently maternally inherited SNHI were identified. In all of these families at least two first-degree relatives with SNHI and with identical mitochondrial genomes were seen.

We found the bp 3243 mutation in five patients suggesting a minimum prevalence of 7.7% in this cohort of maternally inherited SNHI. Three of these patients presented with a multisystem disorder, whereas two had an essentially non-syndromal SNHI. The bp 7445 mutation was not detected in any of the patients.

It is proposed that mitochondrial mutations specify a distinct subtype of SNHI. The total frequency of mitochondrial mutations among patients with SNHI is probably higher than that observed here as only two separate mutations were studied.

PART X
SYNDROMAL CONDITIONS

Chapter 25
Otorhinolaryngological manifestations of Stickler syndrome linked to chromosome 6 near the *COL11A2* gene

RJC ADMIRAAL, HG BRUNNER, PLM HUYGEN and CWRJ CREMERS

Introduction

Stickler syndrome is an autosomal dominant disorder of connective tissue which includes ocular and systemic features. Stickler et al. (1965) described a family with progressive myopia beginning in the first decade of life and resulting in retinal detachment and blindness. Because the affected persons also exhibited premature degenerative changes in various joints with abnormal epiphyseal development and slight hypermobility, the disorder was tentatively termed 'hereditary progressive arthro-ophthalmopathy'. Stickler and Pugh (1967) added radiological abnormalities and sensorineural hearing impairment (SNHI) to the features typical of this syndrome. Hall (1974) pointed out that the Pierre Robin anomaly also forms part of the syndrome, together with typical orofacial features. Hearing impairment was attributed to recurrent otitis media, although SNHI was also described. Hall (1974) concluded that, within a given family, a marked variability in the expression of the gene occurred, both with regard to the severity of involvement and to the organ systems involved. Liberfarb and Goldblatt (1986) found that 50% of females and 43% of males had mitral valve prolapse. Stickler syndrome is nowadays recognized as the most common autosomal dominant connective tissue dysplasia. It includes the features presented in Table 25.1.

Table 25.1 Features of the Stickler syndrome

Ocular	High myopia, vitreoretinal degeneration, retinal detachment, cataract, glaucoma, blindness
Orofacial	Mid-face hypoplasia, micrognathia, cleft/high palate, submucous cleft
Hearing	Conductive and/or SNHI
Cardiac	Mitral valve prolapse
Skeletal	Epiphyseal dysplasia, broad valgus femoral neck, protrusio acetabuli, genu valgus, degenerative arthritis, kyphosis, scoliosis, vertebral disc space narrowing, joint hyperextensibility

Zlogotora et al. (1992) described three families with Stickler syndrome and concluded that the phenotype was variable, but more so *between* than *within* families. Francomano et al. (1986) and Knowlton et al. (1989) found linkage between Stickler syndrome and the type II procollagen locus on chromosome 12, which was further supported by the finding of Ahmad (1990) of a family with a mutation in this gene. In an additional family, however, Bonaventure et al. (1992) excluded linkage to the *COL2A1* gene.

At the moment, it is assumed that in approximately half of the families Stickler syndrome is not linked to *COL2A1*. Brunner et al. (1994) performed linkage analysis in a large Dutch family with Stickler syndrome not linked to the *COL2A1* gene. Close linkage was demonstrated with polymorphic markers at 6p22–p21.3 with a lod score of 4.36. As *COL11A2* has also been localized to this region, it is possible that a mutation in this gene exists in the present family.

Clinical features in the family

In the first, second and third generations, 16 of 20 individuals were affected: all six members in the second generation and nine of 13 persons in the third generation. One patient (III.2) died neonatally from severe asphyxia and aspiration; she had micrognathia and cleft palate.

Facial features included flat mid face and short upturned nose with depressed nasal bridge and protruding eyes. These features were most prominent in childhood and became less obvious with age.

Eleven of 15 affected individuals complained of painful joints. Degenerative changes in spinal and knee joints were documented radiologically in three subjects. All patients had ophthalmological and optometric examinations. Patient II.5 had –3.75 and –4 dioptres myopia, patient II.6 –4.25 and -0.25, and patient III.11 –4.5 in both eyes. Such a moderate myopia cannot be reasonably attributed to the Stickler syndrome. No other affected individuals showed ophthalmological symptoms. The fact that otological and skeletal manifestations occur in this family without ocular involvement might be explained by assuming that the causative mutation is in the *COL11A2* gene, which encodes the α-2 chain of type XI collagen and that the vitreous would not depend on this gene product.

A cleft palate was present in four patients (III.2, III.4, III.7 and III.10). Submucous cleft was present in two cases (II.6 and III.8) and one patient (II.5) showed a high-arched palate.

Hearing loss was noted in all 15 affected persons. One person (III.6) showed an unexplained conductive loss of about 20 dB without otological symptoms. Mixed hearing loss was present in four individuals due to recurrent otitis media, for which ear surgery (tympanoplasty, radical mastoidectomy) was necessary. Two of these patients had a cleft palate and one had a submucous cleft. Thus, three out of five patients with submucous or overt cleft palate showed middle ear disease, whereas only one person out of 10 without cleft palate showed this feature (not significant in Fisher's exact probability test, p (one-tailed) = 0.077). The other 10 patients showed SNHI.

Hearing thresholds (regarding the sensorineural loss or component only) were generally between 30–60 dB in both ears. Analysis of the regression of threshold on age failed to show any significant progression of hearing impairment. Progression was noted in serial audiograms in seven cases but, here too, it was not significant, perhaps because of a lack of sufficient longitudinal data. Considerable variability in the severity of SNHI was noted.

The shape of the audiogram showed the existence of various types, including mid- and high-frequency losses. For the group of affected people as a whole, high-frequency impairments predominated.

Speech audiometry disclosed speech reception thresholds as expected from the pure tone threshold data; a 100% discrimination score was attained in all cases and there was no sign of 'roll-over' (i.e. decrease in discrimination score with increasing stimulus) which might be suggestive of retrocochlear hearing impairment.

Conclusions

We present a family with Stickler syndrome, without ophthalmic involvement, which showed linkage to the *COL11A2* region on 6p22–p21.3. Facial features included flat mid-face, upturned nose with depressed nasal bridge and protruding eyes, and were most prominent in childhood but became less obvious at a more advanced age. Overt cleft palate was present in four individuals and submucous cleft in two (six of 16).

SNHI was generally present with a threshold of between 30–60 dB bilaterally and included mid-frequency loss and predominantly, high-frequency loss. Although serial audiometry was suggestive of progression in some individual cases, a regression analysis of hearing threshold on age at each frequency failed to detect any significant progression in hearing impairment.

Chapter 26
Dominant hemifacial microsomia in a four-generation pedigree

A McINERNEY, R WINTER and M BITNER-GLINDZICZ

Introduction

Various terms have been used to describe this condition — hemifacial microsomia, first and second branchial arch syndrome, oculoauriculovertebral dysplasia and Goldenhar syndrome. Where epibulbar dermoids are present the term 'Goldenhar syndrome' is frequently used but, in their absence and where both sides of the face are affected, the terms 'first' and 'second branchial arch syndrome' may be preferable. Where the face is affected on one side only, without an epibulbar dermoid, the term 'hemifacial microsomia' has been used.

The main features are those of facial asymmetry, small or dysplastic ears (microtia) and preauricular skin tags in a line between the front of the ear and the side of the mouth. Other features include macrostomia, micrognathia, stenosed or atretic external auditory meati, ossicular malformations and more rarely cardiac, renal and vertebral anomalies (hence the term 'oculoauriculovertebral dysplasia').

Most cases are sporadic in nature and recurrence risks are low, although rare dominant families have been reported. We describe here a large four-generation family with remarkable intrafamilial variability and at least two cases of non-penetrance (Figure 26.1).

Case 1

The proband IV-II is a female infant born at term following a normal pregnancy and delivery. She was the first child born to unrelated Caucasian parents, although she had a half-sister by her father's previous relationship. At birth she was noted to have macrostomia, a small jaw, bilateral preauricular skin tags and right microtia with atresia of the right external auditory meatus. In infancy she experienced difficulties

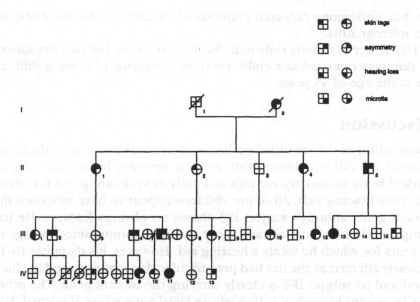

Figure 26.1 Family tree of the extended family.

with feeding, suffered from obstructive sleep apnoea and underwent surgery to advance her jaw. Developmental milestones have been normal but she has some speech delay and, at five years of age, she attends normal school. She has a significant right-sided hearing loss, conductive in nature, and computer tomography (CT) scan shows an absent right external auditory canal and a right hypoplastic middle ear cleft with the malleus fused to a cleft of bone. The inner ear structures are normal. Her heart, kidneys and neck are normal.

Her father was noted to have facial scarring secondary to the removal of preauricular skin tags in childhood. He has facial asymmetry, maxillary hypoplasia and a small jaw. His ears are normal except for narrow external auditory meati. His first child, by a previous partner, is said to have preauricular skin tags but she has not been examined.

Case 2

This girl, III-13, is the first cousin once-removed of Case 1, the proband. She is now aged 18 years. She was the first child born to unrelated Caucasian parents. Pregnancy and delivery were normal. At birth, she had macrostomia, micrognathia, bilateral preauricular skin tags and narrow external auditory meati with asymmetrical involvement of the face. She is developmentally normal and has attended normal school.

She has undergone repeated craniofacial surgery for the macrostomia and micrognathia.

Her father manifests only mild facial asymmetry, but had preauricular skin tags removed as a child. He now complains of hearing difficulties at the age of 45 years.

Discussion

Examination of the extended pedigree shows that many individuals are affected by this condition with varying severity. Individual I-2 had marked facial asymmetry, ear tags and early onset hearing loss for which she wore hearing aids. All of her children appear to have inherited the mutant gene, although subject II-3 shows no obvious features. He has complained of hearing loss and more recently tinnitus since the age of 43 years for which he wears a hearing aid. However, his daughter III-10 is clearly affected as she has had preauricular skin tags removed in childhood and so subject II-3 is clearly carrying the mutant gene. The other non-penetrant individual is III-3 whose facial appearance is normal. Her son IV-5, however, has facial asymmetry, mild bilateral facial weakness but no skin tags, and is likely to be affected.

Several individuals in this pedigree appear to manifest additional features which have been described previously in association with hemifacial microsomia/branchial arch syndrome. Individual III-12 was born with facial asymmetry, preauricular tags and a tracheo-oesophageal fistula (TOF). Her mother, II-4 has preauricular skin tags, facial asymmetry and early onset hearing loss and is therefore a carrier of the mutant gene. The association with TOF has been reported previously which makes it unlikely to be a coincidental occurrence. Sutphen et al., (1995) recently reviewed the association with TOF. In their series, three of 60 patients had TOF or oesophageal atresia (OA). One of their cases was reported to have had severe hearing loss but no details were given.

Affected individual III-2, had a child who died of hydrocephalus. Hydrocephalus has also been recorded previously in patients with this spectrum of branchial arch defects. Schrander-Stumpel et al. (1992) described three cases of the oculoauriculovertebral spectrum and hydrocephalus and reviewed the association. They mentioned that one-third of cases with this combination died early, as in this case. In their review, the children with this association were at increased risk of having cerebral malformations and mental retardation.

Individual IV-13 whose mother, III-7, has facial asymmetry and a history of skin tags, was born with marked plagiocephaly. As IV-13 has no other features of branchial arch syndrome it is difficult to know whether he has inherited the mutant gene from his mother, or whether this is a chance association. A search for radiographic craniosynostosis and extracranial manifestations might indicate whether the plagiocephaly is part of the hemifacial microsomia/oculoauriculovertebral spectrum (Padwa et al., 1993).

Candidate genes have been suggested for hemifacial microsomia. Graham et al. (1995), reported a large family with features of Goldenhar syndrome (with epibulbar dermoids, microtia, micrognathia) and ear tags, ear pits and branchial cysts which maps to 8q11–8q13, the region which harbours the BOR gene. It is not yet known whether the family reported here suffers from an allelic form of branchio–oto–renal (BOR) syndrome, but they do not have epibulbar dermoids or branchial cysts/fistulae.

A second possible candidate gene is the Treacle gene, responsible for cases of the Treacher Collins (mandibulofacial dysosotosis) syndrome. In the first arch mouse mutant, *far*, the phenotype is one of bilateral craniofacial anomalies similar to those seen in Treacher Collins syndrome. This mutation on a different genetic background however can result in a maxillary hemifacial deficiency observed in heterozygotes and it has been postulated that hemifacial and bilateral deficiencies may be due to the same gene (Cousley et al., 1992; Dixon, 1996).

Otological malformations in hemifacial microsomia have been detailed by Phelps (Phelps and Lloyd, 1989). Although the sample would have been biased from the point of view of ascertainment, in few of the 61 temporal bones examined was the middle ear cavity found to be of normal size and shape. The ossicles were found to be frequently absent or abnormal in size, shape and situation. CT scanning of individuals in this family with uninvestigated hearing loss may reveal similar abnormalities.

Linkage studies will indicate whether any of the candidate genes are likely to underlie the condition in this family. If linkage excludes potential candidate regions we plan to conduct a genome search to map the mutant gene.

Conclusions

Hemifacial microsomia is a condition which comprises facial asymmetry, malar hypoplasia, microtia, skin tags and hearing loss. When found in association with an epibulbar dermoid it is termed 'Goldenhar syndrome', and both conditions are usually sporadic in nature, although occasional dominant pedigrees have been reported. In a family with a dominant Goldenhar-like syndrome, linkage has been reported to the BOR syndrome region on 8q. We describe a large four-generation pedigree with dominant inheritance of hemifacial microsomia without epibulbar dermoids in whom there is a highly variable presentation. Penetrance varies considerably ranging from asymptomatic gene carriers (with affected parents and children) to severely affected children with macrostomia, dysplastic or absent external ears, malar hypoplasia, micrognathia and hearing loss (reminiscent of first and second branchial arch syndrome). The associated malformations seen in some individuals in this family are described along with their possible relationship to this condition.

Chapter 27
Variability of expression of sensorineural hearing loss in Usher syndrome: report of a family

D ZANETTI and AR ANTONELLI

Introduction

Congenital hearing impairment may be associated with disorders of other systems and it may be the first symptom of a previously unsuspected syndromal disease (Table 27.1). Ocular involvement is linked to sensorineural hearing impairment (SNHI) in Usher, Cockayne and Lawrence–Moon–Biedl syndromes, and accompanies Refsum and Niemann–Pick diseases.

Usher syndrome (Usher, 1914) is an autosomal recessive disorder, characterized by progressive retinitis pigmentosa (RP) and moderate to severe SNHI. It is estimated to account for 6–10% of all congenital SNHI. Hearing impairment usually precedes the onset of visual symptoms. Electroretinography may be used to identify electrical changes in the eyes prior to any defect being observed with the ophthalmoscope. The absence of cochlear microphonic potentials points to dysfunction of the hair cells as the cause of the hearing impairment.

Recent advances in genetic analysis have been able to identify at least six gene mutations related to Usher syndrome; according to different clinical presentation it has been subtyped in types I, II and III. Early recognition of the syndrome subtype by its phenotypic expression (SNHI, vestibular dysfunction retinal degeneration) is important for counselling and prevention. As already reported in the literature, this is often difficult because of the genetic heterogeneity and variability of phenotypic expression of the disorder, confirmed by the present family screening.

141

Table 27.1 Eye abnormalities associated with hearing impairment*

Syndrome	Characteristics	Mode of inheritance	Type of hearing impairment
Usher	RP, vestibulo-cerebellar ataxia, mental retardation	Recessive	SNHI
Cockayne	Retinal atrophy, motor disturbances, mental retardation, dwarfism	Recessive	SNHI
Alström	Obesity, diabetes mellitus, retinal degeneration	Recessive	SNHI
Halgren	RP, vestibulo-cerebellar ataxia, nystagmus, sometimes mental retardation	Recessive	SNHI
Laurence–Moon–Biedl	RP, polydactyly, hypogenitalism, obesity, mental retardation	Recessive	SNHI
Refsum	RP, cerebellar ataxia, polyneuritis, electrocardiographic abnormalities, ichthyosis-type skin disorder	Recessive	SNHI
Duane	Ocular palsy (congenital fibrous replacement of rectus muscle), auricular malformation, meatal atresia, torticollis, cervical rib, cervical spina bifida	Recessive	Mixed
Moebius	Facial diplegia, lateral and/or medial rectus palsy bilaterally, auricular malformation, micrognathia, absence of hands, feet, fingers or toes, tongue paralysis, mental retardation	Recessive	Mixed

*Modified from Black et al. (1971) Congenital Deafness: A New Approach to Diagnosis Using a High Risk Register. Boulder, CO: Associated University Press.

Material and methods

A 30-year-old female came to observation because of an apparently progressive bilateral SNHI of unknown origin. Her medical history indicated a similar hearing problem in one brother, who had been previously referred for consultation to an ophthalmologist for a visual field defect. After RP was suspected, a detailed pedigree of the family and relatives was obtained (Figure 27.1), and all members underwent an audiological and an ophthalmological screening including:

- Ophthalmoscopy.
- Electroretinography (ERG).
- Complete ENT examination.
- Pure tone audiometry (PTA).
- Middle ear admittance testing.
- Auditory brainstem responses (ABR).
- Vestibular assessment – ENG recording of spontaneous, gaze-evoked and head-shaking nystagmus; caloric tests with the Fitzgerald–Hallpike protocol.

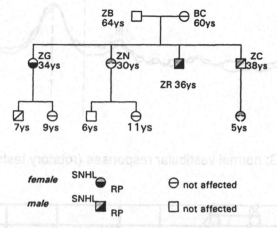

Figure 27.1 Variable phenotypic expression of sensorineural hearing impairment (SNHI) and retinitis pigmentosa (RP) in the family investigated.

Two of the subject's three brothers showed some degree of RP, whereas her fundi were normal.

The subject showed moderate bilateral SNHI (Figure 27.2); her two brothers had a mild high-tone loss and her sister normal hearing. All subjects had normal admittance and ABRs, pointing to cochlear dysfunction.

Vestibular tests were normal in one brother and one sister of the subject; she and the other brother with RP showed bilaterally reduced caloric responses, without significant asymmetry. Both complained of oscillopsia induced by sudden head movement and some difficulty when walking in darkness.

Four out of five children of the three siblings (see Figure 27.1 above) showed no sign of audiological or ocular involvement; one child only had a mild SNHI in the high-frequency range; vestibular testing was not performed on them. No evidence of audio-vestibular or ocular impairment was discovered in either grandparent. The clinical picture is consistent with Usher syndrome type II; further differentiation between types IIA and IIB in relation to linkage to chromosome 1q32–q41 was not possible because the DNA Study was not yet available.

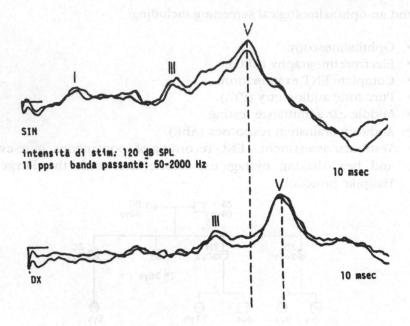

ENG: normal vestibular responses (rotatory tests)

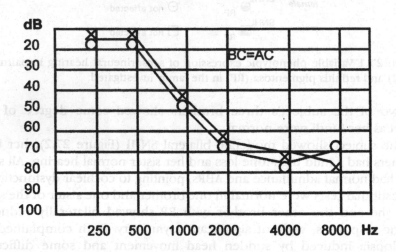

Figure 27.2 Results of otoneurological assessment in the proband.

Discussion

Recent surveys indicate that, in Western countries, approximately 1/1000 children is born deaf. Approximately 50% of all congenital deafness can be attributed to genetic factors, and approximately one-third of hearing impaired children have additional abnormalities (Jacobson,

1995), the majority of which are transmitted through recessive genes. Since for most cases no treatment is available, prevention remains the primary means of reducing the high prevalence of genetic hearing impairment. It can, of course, be accomplished only through genetic counselling of high-risk individuals, i.e. carriers of the gene for deafness.

Identification of the genes is based on linkage analysis (gene localization) and sequencing of the gene itself. By these investigations, it has become apparent that some syndromal SNHI, which had previously been thought of as single entities with a variable range of expression, were, in fact, more than one entity, linked to unrelated sections of chromosomes. This is the case with Usher syndrome, which has been classified as types I, II and III, according to different clinical presentations; at least six USH loci have been identified to date (Table 27.2).

Table 27.2 Clinical features of Usher syndrome subtypes

Subtype	Hearing loss	Retinitis pigmentosa	Vestibular responses	Mapped genes
I	Severe to profound	Present in childhood	Absent or reduced	14q31; 11q13.5; 1p13–15
II	Moderate to severe	Present, late onset	Normal	1q41
III	Variable	Present at any age	?	3q

The main clinical features of Usher syndrome are progressive RP and congenital moderate to severe SNHI. Inheritance of this disease is autosomal recessive. The visual field is gradually constricted as pigment deposits occur in the periphery of the retina. Two of the three brothers of the reported family showed some degree of RP. Cataracts may also occur. The clinical manifestations include a range of psychological–emotional disorders for which psychological testing and counselling is recommended.

In Usher syndrome type I the hearing impairment is usually bilateral and severe. In types II and III it is milder (see Table 27.2). The pathological condition of the cochlea tends to be of the Alexander type, that is an end-organ lesion in the basal turn of an otherwise normal membranous labyrinth (Belal, 1975). Our subject showed moderate to severe bilateral SNHI (see Figure 27.2); her brothers had a mild high-tone loss and her sister normal hearing.

Diagnosis relies primarily upon a thorough medical history and examination. The association with RP is rarely discovered at the time of the confirmation of the SNHI, because it is not found at fundoscopy in childhood and does not cause visual problems until later in infancy.

Electroretinography (ERG) can disclose signs of retinal damage prior to their clinical manifestation, but its value as a routine investigation is controversial. In the present series, it helped identify electrical changes in the eyes before any defect was observed with the ophthalmoscope in two cases (Figure 27.3).

Common causes of SNHI, such as noise or mechanical trauma, drug ototoxicity, infections etc., must be excluded. Full audiological assessment follows, including pure tone and speech audiometry (articulation curve), middle ear impedance testing and recording of ABR. All tests gave normal results in the family investigated, except for abnormal latencies of ABR peaks in the proband. Electrocochleography shows an absence of cochlear microphonics (Abraham et al., 1977) and Békésy audiometry has shown excellent specificity but poor sensitivity (Kloepfer et al., 1966); these tests were not performed in the present study. Abnormal or absent vestibular responses are frequent (Bellman, 1987) but not diagnostic; they can identify a higher risk group; our proband showed bilaterally reduced vestibular responses, whereas all her relatives had normal labyrinthine function.

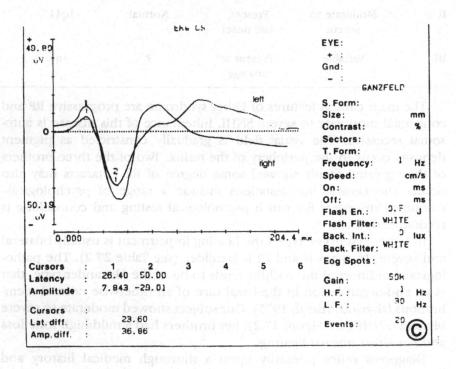

Figure 27.3 ERG helped to disclose signs of retinal damage before any defect was observed with the ophthalmoscope.

Differential diagnosis includes other syndromes with ocular involvement, such as mandibulo-facial dysostosis, in which microtia and micrognathia are evident, and Kearns–Sayre syndrome, associated with brain and multiple organ abnormalities (see Table 27.1).

Genetic linkage analysis requires the availability of research facilities and good cooperation with laboratory investigators. Investigation of the family pedigree is of utmost importance, and ophthalmologic consultation is needed in every family member to detect the of RP.

Parental counselling is important to enable parents to make informed reproductive choices; in the non-hearing population, for instance, marriage of two individuals with different mutations (aa × bb) carries a negligible risk, while consanguinuity is a critical factor. A detailed estimate of the individual probability of siblings expressing the disease has been calculated by some authors (Ruben and Rapin, 1988; Dallapiccola et al., 1996). Empirically, when a child has a profound SNHI, the risk of a second child being affected is 1:6.

When SNHL is recognized, rehabilitation should be started immediately. Therefore, it is important that the otologist be alert to the possibility of other defects associated with the deafness. Our subject showed severe bilateral SNHI and a pathological retina on examination; RP was diagnosed in two of her three siblings by ERG; one brother had a mild high-tone loss and her sister normal hearing.

The inconstant manifestation of both SNHI and RP in this family confirms the variability of phenotypic expression of the disease already reported in the literature (Larget-Pier et al., 1994; Gorlin et al., 1995).

Pieke Dahl et al. (1993) reported a family with clinical Usher syndrome type II (but with milder SNHI and vestibular involvement) not linked with the already recognized USH genes. The authors pointed out that this genetic heterogeneity limits the possibility of early identification based on phenotypic characteristics.

The present report adds further evidence of this variable clinical expression of Usher syndrome type II, and stresses the need for a genetic linkage analysis.

Chapter 28
Mpv17 — Glomerulosclerosis gene is essential for inner ear function

AM MEYER ZUM GOTTESBERGE, B ESCHEN, A REUTER,
L KINTRUP and H WEIHER

Introduction

The Mpv17 mouse strain is characterized by the development of early onset glomerulosclerosis (Weiher et al., 1990) and, as found recently, by impairment of the inner ear function (Meyer zum Gottesberge et al., 1996). The phenotype results from loss of function of a gene coding for a 20 kDa hydrophobic peroxisomal protein of 176 amino acids, which was destroyed by a retroviral integration (Zwacka et al., 1994). The nephrotic syndrome shows characteristic changes of physiological parameters in serum, blood and urine. The serum changes include elevation of urea levels, as well as of creatinine and cholesterol levels. Furthermore, in end-stage disease, severe proteinuria as well as anaemia occur. Histologically, the picture is of focal segmental glomerulosclerosis.

The human homologue of the Mpv17 gene has been isolated and studied (Karasawa et al., 1993). It is structurally highly homologous to the mouse gene (>92% at the protein level) and can, if introduced into the mutant mice as a transgene, rescue the phenotype (Schenkel et al., 1995). However, until now no defects in the Mpv17 gene have been found associated with familial cases of glomerulosclerosis.

In a preliminary report we have documented major morphological alterations including degeneration of the stria vascularis and spiral ligament, loss of cochlear neurones and degeneration of the organ of Corti in the Mpv17 mice (Meyer zum Gottesberge et al., 1996). In order to extend this study, a detailed light, transmission and scanning electron microscopic analysis was performed, showing changes reminiscent of those reported for Alport syndrome in man (Weidauer and Arnold, 1976; Arnold, 1984). Alport syndrome is an inherited disorder characterized by progressive nephritis and neurosensory deafness (Atkin,

1988). Although the molecular defect is of a different nature from that in Alport patients (Tryggvason et al., 1993), we believe that studying the pathogenic mechanisms in Mpv17 mice might help to elucidate the pathological processes in the human disease, in particular the relationship between the kidney and inner ear.

Material and method

Twenty-five Mpv17 transgenic mice and 15 control mice (CFW mice) of both sexes, aged between 2–18 months were used in this study. The animals were anaesthetized with ether and perfused through the aorta with rinse solution (containing NaCl, procaine, polyvinyl-pyrrolidone and heparin, pH 7.3), followed by a cacodylate-buffered solution containing 2.5% glutaraldehyde fixative, pH 7.3 for 5 min. Alternatively, the animals were decapitated, the bullae removed and the cochleae exposed. Fresh fixative, equilibrated at room temperature before use, was carefully injected into the cochlea through an opening in the apex and oval window. The bullae were removed and fixed for 24 h at 4°C. One side was decalcified in 10% EDTA, post-fixed in 1% cacodylate-buffered OsO_4 for 1 h at room temperature, dehydrated and embedded in Epon resin and sectioned parallel to the modiolus. Scanning electron microscopy was used to evaluate the loss of the hair cells. The other cochleae were post-fixed in 1% cacodylate-buffered OsO_4 for 1 h at room temperature, dehydrated to 70% ethanol before dissection, finally dehydrated through acetone and dried in a critical point dryer. Kidneys were removed and immersed in 2.5% glutaraldehyde in cacodylate buffer, pH 7.3, for 24 h, post-fixed in 1% cacodylate buffered OsO_4 for 1 h at room temperature, dehydrated with ethanol and embedded in Epon resin.

Results

Histological study of the inner ears of Mpv17 mice revealed degeneration of the stria vascularis and spiral ligament, loss of cochlear neurons and degeneration of the organ of Corti. These changes were present in both female and male animals, but were more prominent in males. We found focal lesions of the stria morphology with radial segmental participation of the organ of Corti and spiral ganglion. The alterations ranged from thinning of the epithelium and absence of capillaries and strial cells, to variation in the size of capillary profiles (Figure 28.1). Ultrastructurally, the changes in the stria vascularis ranged from a decrease in the extent of the basal foldings of the marginal cells and its degeneration, to complete disintegration and atrophy of the strial epithelium (Figure 28.2).

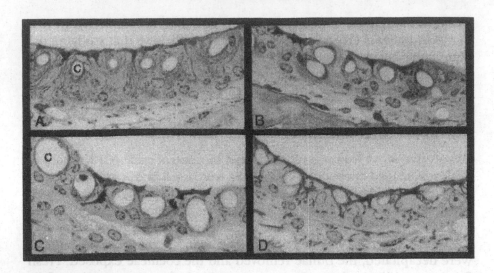

Figure 28.1 Semi-thin section of the stria vascularis showing variation of the pathomorphology, including the size of the capillaries and strial epithelium and its organization, within cochlea of Mpv17 mice. (A) apex; (B) upper middle turn; (C) lower middle turn; (D) basal turn of same cochlea (male, 7 months old); c = capillary; magnification 700×.

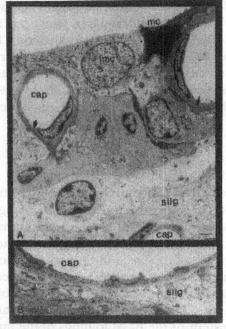

Figure 28.2 Electron micrograph of the lateral wall of the Mpv17 mouse cochlea showing reorganization of the strial epithelium and thickening of the capillary basal lamina (arrow) of the stria vascularis in contrast to spiral ligament. (A) stria vascularis and spiral ligament; (B) spiral ligament; cap = capillary; imc = intermedial cells; mc = marginal cell; slig = spiral ligament; bar = 1 μm.

The basal infolding of the marginal cells appeared condensed and surrounded by electron dense material. There were, however, considerable variations in the pathology, the lesions had progressed further in older animals and they appeared more severe compared with age-matched control subjects. The most common and prominent finding for all Mpv17 mice was alteration of the basement membrane of the strial capillary (Figure 28.3). The basal lamina was thickened and showed fragmentation or splitting. In contrast, the capillary wall of the spiral ligament showed a normal appearance (Figure 28.2).

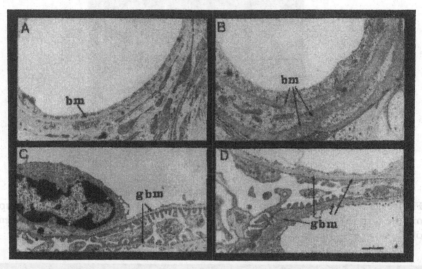

Figure 28.3 Higher magnification of the strial capillary wall (A, B) and the glomerular epithelial and endothial cells (C, D) reveal perivascular thickening of the basement membrane (arrow) in Mpv17 versus control mice. Ultrastructural characteristics of the glomeruli are depicted in C (control) and D (Mpv17) showing the thickness of the glomerular basement membrane, irregularity of the epithelial side and the fusion of the epithelial foot processes. bm = strial basement membrane; gbm = glomerular basement membrane; Bar = 1 μm.

The spiral prominentia was less affected in most cases, although in some specimens it could be seen to have degenerated. Atrophy of the spiral ligament was associated with disorientation of the collageneous fibres and decrease of stromal cell number. The organ of Corti appeared collapsed, there was frequently loss of the outer hair cells and occasionally inner hair cells were missing (Figure 28.4). There were great variations in the morphology of the organ of Corti, ranging from partly damaged receptor cells with all cell types of the organ of Corti still recognisable, to the presence of only a low undifferentiated epithelium covering the basilar membrane. The Mpv17 strain showed an atrophy of spiral ganglion cells and reduced nerve fibres in regions with impaired hair cells (Figure 28.5), often with affected stria vascularis. Degenerative changes in the glomerular visceral epithelial cells, enlarged glomerular basement membrane with electron dense material deposited in the subendothelial space were observed in the kidney of Mpv17 mice, therefore corroborating earlier data.

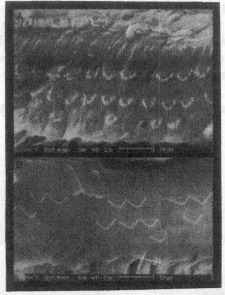

Figure 28.4 Scanning electron microscopical view of organ of Corti from the upper middle turn (A) and basal turn (B) of the Mpv17 mouse. Note the increased number of missing outer hair cells in the basal turn.

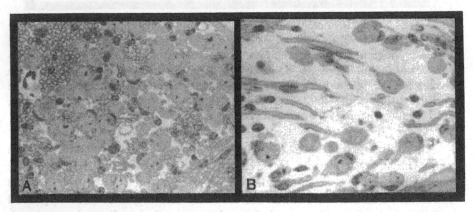

Figure 28.5 Semi-thin section of the spiral ganglion and nerve fibres in the middle turn (A) control, (B) Mpv17 mouse. Magnification 640×.

Discussion

Clinical and experimental data show that there is a strong relationship between the kidney and the inner ear. Because of the morphological similarities, the often concurrent ototoxicity and nephrotoxicity of aminoglycosides and the coexisting congenital anomalies in the kidney and inner ear (reviewed in Schuknecht 1973; Arnold and Friedmann, 1992), Quick et al. (1973) and Arnold et al. (1976) suggested that a common structural basis or shared antigenic determinants of these two organs may be a cause of these disorders. Failure to express the Mpv17 gene causes a phenotype of glomerulosclerosis and nephrotic syndrome and, as demonstrated in this study, an alteration of inner ear structures which leads to hearing impairment. The abnormalities of the stria vascularis were concurrent with alterations of the organ of Corti and the spiral ganglion. The structural abnormalities were observed in both young and older animals, although they were more prominent in the older ones, so it is not possible to determine whether the stria vascularis and the hair cells were affected sequentially or in parallel. To clarify this more detailed studies are required. However, it seems that changes of the basement membrane of the capillary in the stria vascularis occur early in the sequential (radial) progression of damage of the cochlea. The finding of a disintegration of the strial epithelium also opens the possibility that this lesion may be caused by a developmental defect. The morphological alterations were present in both females and males, but they were more prominent in males. The stria vascularis appeared thinner. A similar thinning was noted by Steel et al. (1987) and by Schrott and Spoendlin (1987) in the white spotting mutant mice which show cochleo-saccular defects. However, unlike in the white spotting mutant, this is not due to missing intermediate cells (melanocytes). The intermediate cells are present in Mpv17 mice but they do not develop dendrites and might be functionally impaired.

In the adult male animals analysed here, there is a definite gradient in the structure of the organ of Corti along the cochlear duct. Often at the base there is only a low undifferentiated epithelium, while at the apex all cell types of the organ of Corti, except for partly damaged receptor cells, are recognizable. The basal to apical gradient in the integrity of the organ of Corti and spiral ganglion is consistent with the pattern generally found in degenerative mutants (Webster, 1985). However, we also found cases in which the lesion of the cochlea, which involved the lateral wall, organ of Corti, and spiral ganglion, was limited to particular parts of the cochlea (focal), independent of the position (basal or apical turn). The appearance of focal lesions in the cochlea is in agreement with the pathological findings in the kidney where focal segmental lesions have also been described in these animals (Weiher, 1993).

The genetic mutation which gives rise to an albino animal has several well known phenotypic characteristics, including a decrease in visual acuity attributed to the absence of melanin (Jacobson et al., 1984). The stria vascularis is also devoid of pigment in albino animals; it contains only unpigmented melanocytes. However, the presence or absence of melanin appeared to have no effect on cochlear degeneration in the aged cochlea (Keithley et al., 1992). One of the consistent features of the aged cochlea is strial degeneration (Cratton and Schulte, 1995). Wild type (control) and Mpv17 mice are albino; the wild type showed some age-related alterations; however, the changes observed in Mpv17 mice were characteristic and present at an early age.

The morphological alterations observed in the Mpv17 mice are similar to those described in a hereditary kidney disorder associated with hearing impairment, Alport syndrome. This is a hereditary disorder characterized by progressive nephritis with ultrastructural changes of the glomerular basement membrane and neurosensory deafness (Atkin, 1988). A variety of pathological findings were described at the light microscopic level: degeneration of the stria vascularis; atrophy of the spiral ganglia and acoustic nerve; vesicle formation in the spiral ligament; loss of hair cells; changes in the supporting cells; and occasionally atrophy of the cristae (reviewed by Schuknecht, 1973; Arnold and Friedmann, 1992). The variability of the findings and the fact that at this time a consistent picture of the inner ear pathology in Alport syndrome does not exist may be due to post-mortem autolysis and fixation artifacts. The pathology of the kidney, easily confirmed by renal biopsy, usually shows thinning and thickening and splitting of the glomerular basement membrane into thin layers and accumulating electron dense particles (Atkin, 1988).

Several types of Alport syndrome, autosomal and X-linked, with and without hearing impairment and ocular lesions have been classified (Atkin, 1988). Clinical features suggested an obvious class of candidate genes related to the glomerular basement membrane whose major components are glycoproteins, collagen IV and laminin. The kidney (Kafalides, 1971) and inner ear (Takahoshi and Hokunan, 1992; Cosgrove et al., 1996) are prominent sites of expression of type IV collagen. Mutations in the genes encoding the different chains of type IV collagen have been found in patients with Alport syndrome. Mutations in the COL4A5 gene encoding the type IV collagen α5 chain have been reported in patients with the X-linked form (Tryggvason et al., 1993), whereas in the autosomal form mutations in the COL4A3 and COL4A4 genes on chromosome 2q were seen (Mochizuki et al., 1994).

A gene mutation in the transgenic mouse Mpv17 causes nephrotic syndrome (Weiher et al., 1990) and leads to a significant alteration of the inner ear structures (Meyer zum Gottesberge et al., 1996), which are directly or indirectly involved in the transduction of sound. It affects the sensory neuroepithelium, the organ of Corti, spiral ganglion cells and the stria vascularis. The stria vascularis is responsible for maintaining the characteristic ionic composition of the endolymph with high K^+ and low Na^+ and generating the unusually high extracellular resting potential, the endocochlear potential (EP), which acts essentially as a driving force for the transduction process. Since this gene defect significantly alters the inner ear structure it was suggested that Mpv17 mice would show a hearing defect at young age. Recently in cooperation with Department of Physiology of the University of Frankfurt we have shown that this assumption is correct (Müller et al., in press).

Genetic factors are likely to play a role in the susceptibility to hearing loss later in life, and understanding how a single gene mutation can cause hearing impairment should help to elucidate the interactions between genetic predisposition and environment which may result in hearing impairment which starts in childhood or in adults. Several genes responsible for late-onset hearing impairment have been identified (reviewed by Steel and Brown, 1994). The Mpv17 gene may be a further candidate for late-onset hearing impairment in man. The Mpv17 gene is well conserved across species and maps in mice to chromosome 5 and in humans to chromosome 2 at band 2p23–21 (Karasawa et al., 1993). Interestingly, Chaib et al. (1996b) recently described a non-syndromal recessive sensorineural hearing impairment gene that maps to 2p22–23.

Conclusions

The Mpv17 mouse strain is a recessive transgenic mouse mutant which develops glomerulosclerosis and nephrotic syndrome at a young age. The phenotype results from loss of function of a gene coding for a 20 kDa hydrophobic peroxisomal protein of 176 amino acids, following its disruption by retroviral integration. To investigate a potential effect of the missing Mpv17 function on the inner ear, light and electron microscopic investigations were performed on the inner ears of Mpv17 mice and controls. Our study has demonstrated that Mpv17-protein is essential for inner ear function and that its deficiency leads to significant morphologically identifiable abnormalities of the inner ear structures which include degeneration of the stria vascularis and spiral ligament, loss of cochlear neurones and degeneration of the organ of Corti. The alterations observed here were similar to those described for Alport syndrome, an inherited disorder characterized by progressive nephritis and neurosensory deafness. These findings indicate that although the molecular cause is different, the Mpv17 mouse model may share pathological mechanisms involved in patients with Alport syndrome. At present the Mpv17 mouse appears to be a suitable animal model for this disorder and may help to further elucidate the relationship between the kidney and the inner ear.

Chapter 29
Cloning of a candidate gene for hearing defects in CATCH 22 syndrome

A PIZZUTI, G NOVELLI, A RATTI, F AMATI, A MARI,
G CALABRESE, S NICOLIS, V SILANI, B MARINO,
G SCARLATO, S OTTOLENGHI, R MINGARELLI and
B DALLAPICCOLA

Abstract

The acronym CATCH 22 (Cardiac defects, Abnormal facies, Thymic hypoplasia, Cleft palate and Hypocalcaemia on chromosome 22) has been proposed to encompass a wide spectrum of clinical manifestations which include conotruncal cardiac malformations, psychiatric disorders, ocular abnormalities, upper-limb malformations, renal and urological tract malformations, cerebellar atrophy, dysmorphic ears and conductive hearing impairment. Hearing defects in CATCH 22 patients vary from normal to profound hearing impairment, and may manifest sensorineural, conductive, or mixed hearing impairment of varying degree. CATCH 22 patients with hearing impairment frequently show cochlear hypoplasia and dysplasia (with Mondini's aplasia), sensory ganglia hypoplasia, absence and defective innervation of the semicircular canals, cristae, saccular hypoplasia, and reduced numbers of ganglionic neurones. Although it seems likely that clinical abnormalities observed in these patients have a common aetiology, none of the genes isolated from the critical region, seems at present to possess the characteristics to determine the constellation of the CATCH 22 defects (Dallapiccola et al., 1996b).

We have now cloned from the CATCH 22 critical region a gene which is expressed early in the otocyst and in other tissues including the trachea and cardiac outflow tract, common targets of the condition. This gene (*UFD1L*) appears to be a homologue of a gene identified in yeast belonging to the ubiquitin fusion protein degradation pathway. This gene was mapped to chromosome 22 by use of FISH analysis in the region frequently deleted in patients with CATCH 22. The expression pattern of the murine *UFD1L* orthologue, *Ufd1l*, suggests a role in the development of most of the components of the inner and middle ear, from the emergence of the otic placode. In the developing cardiac structure, the expression pattern is indicative of a role for *Ufd1l* in the cardiac outflow tract. Assuming a similar pattern of expression of the human orthologue during development, these mutiple sites of expression could thus account for the ear anomalies of CATCH 22 syndrome (Baxter et al., 1993; Smith-Thomas et al., 1994).

Mammalian cells contain multiple proteolytic systems, including the ubiquitin-proteasome pathway (Mitch et al., 1996). The ubiquitin–proteasome pathway is considered the most efficient and selective intracellular system for protein degradation which appears to be essential for the control of growth and metabolism during development (Mitch et al., 1996). Ubiquitination is important for inner ear development as suggested by elevated ubiquitin C-terminal hydrolase levels in non-neuronal cochlea cells from its early development, persisting until after hearing has commenced (Smith-Thomas et al., 1994). It is therefore plausible that a reduction in activity of the *UFD1L* gene can affect the normally rapid degradation of proteins, impairing the adaptation to new physiological conditions of neural crest cells during differentiation. In conclusion, the haploinsufficiency of *UFD1L* observed in CATCH 22 syndrome is indicative of a crucial role of the ubiquitin proteasome pathway in developmental processes.

Acknowledgement

This work was supported by grants from Italian Telethon and MURST.

References

Abraham FA, Cohen D and Sohmer H. (1977) Usher's syndrome: electrophysiological test of the visual and auditory systems. Documenta Ophthalmologica 44: 435–44.

Ahmad NN, Ala-Kokko L, Knowlton RG, Weaver EJ, Maguire JI, Tasman W and Procktop DJ. (1990) A stop codon in the gene for type II collagen (COL2A1) causes one variant of arthro-ophthalmopathy (the Stickler syndrome). American Journal of Human Genetics 47: A206.

Alexander G. (1904) Zur Pathologie und pathologischen Anatomie der kongenitalen Taubheit. Archiv fur Klinische und Experimentelle Ohren-, Nasan- und Kehlkopfheilkunde 61: 183–219.

Alksne LE, Anthony RA, Liebman SW and Warner JR. (1993) An accuracy center in the ribosome conserved over 2 billion years. Proceedings of the National Academy of Sciences 90: 9538–41.

Anderson K and Wedenberg E. (1968) Audiometric identification of normal hearing carriers of genes for deafness. Acta Otolaryngologica 65: 535–54.

Arnold W. (1984) Inner ear and renal diseases. Annals of Otology Rhinology and Laryngology 93: 119–23.

Arnold W and Friedmann I. (1992) Pathology of the Inner Ear. London: Churchill Livingstone.

Arnold W, Weidauer H and Seelig HP. (1976) Experimenteller Beweis einer gemeinsamen Antigenizität zwischen Innenohr und Niere. Archives of Otorhinolaryngology 212: 99–117.

Arslan E, Trevisi P, Genovese E, Lupi G and Prosser S. (1991) Hearing loss aetiology in a group of 996 children. Annals of the New York Academy of Sciences 630: 315.

Atkin CL, Gregory MC and Border WA. (1988) Alport syndrome. In: Schrier RW, Gotschalk CS (eds), Diseases of the Kidney. Boston, MA: Little, Brown, pp. 617–41.

Baldwin CT, Farrer LA, Weiss S, De Stefano AL, Adair R, Franklyn B, Kidd KK, Korostishevsky M and Bonné-Tamir B. (1995) Linkage of congenital, recessive deafness (DFNB4) to chromosome 7q31 and evidence for genetic heterogenecity in the Middle Eastern Druze population. Human Molecular Genetics 4: 1637–42.

Ballinger SW, Shoffner JH, Hedaya EV et al. (1992) Maternally transmitted diabetes and deafness associated with a 10.4 kb mitochondrial DNA deletion. Nature and Genetics 1: 11–15.

Barba D, Hardin J, Ray J and Gage FH. (1993) Thyidine kinase-mediated killing of rat brain tumors. Journal of Neurosurgery 79: 729–35.

Baxter R, Bannister LH, Dodson HC and Gathercole DV. (1993) Protein gene product 9.5 in the developing cochlea of the rat: cellular distribution and relation to the cochlear cytoskeleton. Journal of Neurocytology 22: 14–25.

Beighton P and Sellars S. (1982) Genetics and Otology. Edinburgh: Churchill Livingstone, p. 80.

Bellman SC. (1987) Hearing disorders in children. British Medical Bulletin 43: 966–82.

Ben Arab S, Bonaiti-Pellié C and Belkahia A. (1990) An epidemiological and genetic study of congenital profound deafness in Tunisia (governorate of Nabeul). Journal of Medical Genetics 27: 29–33.

Berkener JK. (1992) Expression of heterologous sequences in adenoviral vectors. Current Topics in Microbiology and Immunology 158: 39–66.

Bergstrom L. (1977) Osteogenesis imperfecta: otologic and maxillofacial aspects. Laryngoscope 7 (Suppl. 6): 1–42.

Bonaventure J, Philippe C, Plessis G, Vigneron J, Lasselin C, Maroteaux P and Gilgenkrantz S. (1992) Linkage study in a large pedigree with Stickler syndrome: exclusion of COL2A1 as the mutant gene. Human Genetics 90: 164–8.

Bonfils P, Avan P, Londero A, Narcy P and Trotoux J. (1991) Progressive hereditary deafness with predominant inner hair cell loss. American Journal of Otology 12: 3–7.

Boviatsis EJ et al. (1994) Gene transfer into experimental brain tumors mediated by adenovirus, herpes simplex virus, and retrovirus vectors. Human Gene Therapy 5: 183–91.

Brody SL and Crystal RG. (1994) Adonovirus-mediated in vivo gene transfer. Annals of the New York Academy of Sciences 716: 90–101.

Brunner HG, van Beersum SEC, Warman ML, Olsen BR, Ropers H-H and Mariman ECM. (1994) Stickler syndrome gene is linked to chromosome 6 near the COL11A2 gene. Human Molecular Genetics 3: 1561–4.

Bu X, Shohat M, Jaber L and Rotter JI. (1993) A form of sensorineural deafness is determined by a mitochondrial and an autosomal locus: evidence from pedigree segregation analysis. Genetic Epidemiology 10: 3–15.

Buetow KH, Weber JL, Ludwigsen S, Scherpbier-Heddema T, Duyk GM, Sheffield VC, Wang Z and Murray JC. (1994) Integrated human genome-wide maps constructed using the CEPH reference panel. Nature Genetics 6: 391–3

Chaib H, Place C, Salem N, Dode C, Chardenoux S, Weissenbach J, El-Zir E, Loiselet J and Petit C. (1996a) Mapping of DFNB12, a gene for non-syndromal autosomal recessive deafness, to chromosome 10q21–22. Human Molecular Genetics 5: 1061–4.

Chaib H, Place CH, Salem N, Chardenoux S, Vincent CH, Weissenbach J, El-Zir E, Loiselt J and Petit CH. (1996b) A gene responsible for a sensorineural nonsyndromic recessive deafness maps to chromosome 2p22–23. Human Molecular Genetics 5: 155–8.

Chaib H, Kaplan J, Gerber S, Vincent C, Ayadi H, Slim R, Munnich A, Weissenbach J and Petit C. (1997) A newly identified locus for Usher Syndrome, USH1E, maps to chromosome 21q21. Human Molecular Genetics 6: 27–31.

Chen A, Francis M, Li N, Cremers CW, Kimberling WJ, Sato Y, Phelps PD, Bellman SC, Wagner MJ and Pembrey M. (1995) Phenotypic manifestations of branchio-oto-renal syndrome. American Journal of Medical Genetics 58: 365–70.

Chomyn A and Attardi G. (1987) Mitochondrial gene products. Current Topics in Bioenergetics 15: 295–329.

Chung CS and Brown KS. (1970) Family studies of early childhood deafness ascertained through the Clarke School for the Deaf. American Journal of Human Genetics 22: 630–44.

Chung CS, Robinson OW and Morton NE. (1959) A note on deaf-mutism. Annals of Human Genetics 23: 357–66.

Cianfaloni E, Ricci E and Shanske S et al. (1992) MELAS: clinical features, biochemistry and molecular genetics. Annals of Neurology 14: 391–8.

Clementi M and Tenconi R. (1994) Etiologia delle ipoacusie preverbali. Audiologia Italiana 11: 10.

Cock E. (1838) The pathology of congenital deafness. Guy's Hospital Reports No. 7: 289–307.

Cohen M, Francis M, Luxon LM, Bellman S, Coffey R and Pembrey M. (1996a) Dips on Békésy or audioscan fail to identify carriers of autosomal recessive non-syndromic hearing loss. Acta Otolaryngologica 116: 521–27.

Cohen M, Prasher DK, Luxon LM, Bellman S and Pembrey M. (1996b) Otoacoustic emissions in obligate carriers of autosomal recessive non-syndromic hearing loss. Abstract. XXIII International Congress of Audiology, Bari.

Cohen-Haguenauer O. (1994) A review of current basic approaches to gene therapy. Nouvelle Revue Française d' Hématologie 36 (Suppl. 1): S3–S9.

Collet L, Veuillet E, Berger-Vachon C and Morgon A. (1992) Evoked otoacoustic emissions: relative importance of age, gender and sensorineural hearing loss using a mathematical model of the audiogram. International Journal of Neuroscience 62: 113–22.

Cosgrove D, Samuelson G and Pinnt J. (1996) Immunohistochemical localization of basement membrane collagens and associated proteins in the murine cochlea. Hearing Research 97: 54–65.

Costeff H and Dar H. (1980) Consanguinity analysis of congenital deafness in northern Israel. American Journal of Human Genetics 32: 64–8.

Coucke P, Van Camp G, Djoyodiharjo B, Oostra B, Huizing EH, Padberg G, Cremers C, Frants R, Van de Heyning PH and Willems P. (1994) Linkage of ausomal dominant hearing loss to the short arm of chromosome 1 in two families. New England Journal of Medicine 331: 425–431.

Cournoyer D and Caskey C. (1993) Gene therapy of the immune system. Annual Review of Immunology 11: 297–329.

Cousley RRJ and Wilson DJ. (1992) Hemifacial microsomia: developmental consequences of perturbation of the auriculofacial cartilage model? American Journal of Medical Genetics 42: 461–6.

Cratton MA and Schulte BA. (1995) Alterations in microvasculature are associated with atrophy of the stria vascularis in quiet-aged gerbils. Hearing Research 82: 44-52.

Dallapiccola B and Mingarelli R et al. (1996a) Aspetti genetici della sordità. Acta Otorhinologica Italiàna 16: 79–90.

Dallapiccola B, Pizzuti A and Novelli G. (1996b) How many breaks do we need to CATCH on 22q11? American Journal of Human Genetics 59: 7–11.

D'Amico A, Brai M, Crino' S and Grisanti G. (1993) An informatic tool for diagnosis of hereditary deafness. Phisica Medica, IX (Suppl. 1): 33–36.

Das VK. (1988) Aetiology of bilateral sensorineural deafness in children. Scandinavian Audiology (Suppl.) 30: 43–52.

David G, Valentino G and Previtero G. (1992) Studio epidemiologico dei deficit uditivi in Avellino e provincia nel decennio 1980–1990. Audiologia Italiana 9: 218–222.

Davidson J, Hyde ML and Aberti PW. (1988) Epidemiology of hearing impairment in childhood. Scandinavian Audiology 30: 13–20.

Davies E, Gladstone HB, Williams H, Hradek G, Shah SB and Schindler RA. (1994) A model for long-term intracochlear administration of pharmacologic agents. American Journal of Otology 15: 757–61.

Deol MS. (1956) The anatomy and development of the mutants pirouette, shaker-1 and waltzer in the mouse. Proceedings of the Royal Society 145: 206–13.

Deol MS and Robins MW. (1962) The spinner mouse. Journal of Heredity 53: 133–6.

Dias O and Andrea M. (1990) Childhood deafness in Portugal: aetiological factors and diagnosis of hearing loss. International Journal of Pediatric Otorhinolaryngology 18: 247.

DiMauro S, Bonilla E, Zeviani M, Nakagawa M and De Vivo DC. (1985) Mitochondrial myopathies. Annals of Neurology 17: 521–38.

Dixon MJ. (1996) Treacher Collins syndrome. Human Molecular Genetics 5: 1391–6.

Dorudi S, Northover J and Vile R. (1993) Gene transfer therapy in cancer. British Journal of Surgery 80: 566–72.

Dunbar DR, Moonie PA, Swingler RJ, Davidson D, Roberts R and Holt IJ. (1993) Maternally transmitted partial direct tandem duplication of mitochondrial DNA associated with diabetes mellitus. Human Molecular Genetics 2: 1619–24.

Dunbar DR, Moonie PA, Zeviani M and Holt IJ. (1996) Complex I deficiency is associated with 3243G:C mitochondrial DNA in oesteosarcoma cell hybrids. Human Molecular Genetics 5: 123–9.

Dunnet S and Svendsen C. (1993) Huntington's disease: animal models and transplantation repair. Current Opinion in Neurobiology 3: 790–6.

Engel JE and Wu CF. (1994) Altered mechanoreceptor responses in Drosophilia bang-sensitive mutants. Behavioural Physiology 175: 267–78.

Enriquez JA, Chomyn A and Attardi G. (1995) mtDNA mutation in MERRF syndrome causes defective aminoacylation of tRNA(lys) and premature translation termination. Nature Genetics 10: 47–55.

Fischel-Ghodsian N, Prezant TR, Fournier P, Stewart IA and Maw M. (1995) Mitochondrial mutation associated with non-syndromic deafness. American Journal of Otolaryngology 16: 403–8.

Fisch L (1981) Syndromes associated with hearing loss. In Beagley HA (ed) Audiology and Audiological Medicine. Oxford: Oxford University Press pp595–639.

Francomano CA, Le P-L, Liberfarb R, Streeten E and Pyeritz RE. (1986) Collagen gene linkage analysis in the Marfan and Stickler syndromes. (Abstract). American Journal of Human Genetics 39: A92.

Fraser GR. (1965) Sex-linked recessive congenital deafness and the excess of males in profound childhood deafness. Annals of Human Genetics 29: 171–96.

Fraser GR. (1976) The Causes of Profound Deafness in Childhood. Baltimore, MD: Johns Hopkins University Press.

French BA. (1993) Gene transfer and cardiovascular disorders. Herz 18: 222–9.

Friedman TB, Liang Y, Weber JL, Hinnant JT, Barber TD, Winata S, Arhya IN and Asher JH Jr. (1995) A gene for congenital, recessive deafness DFNB3 maps to the pericentromeric region of chromosome 17. Nature and Genetics 9: 86–91.

Froidevaux S and Loor F. (1991) A quick procedure for identifying doubly homozygous immunodeficient scid beige mice. Journal of Immunological Methods 137: 275–9.

Fukushima K, Arabandi R, Srisailapathy CRS, Ni L, Chen A, O'Neill M, Van Camp G, Coucke P, Smith SD, Kenyon JB, Jain P, Wilcox ER, Zbar RIS and Smith RJH. (1995a) Consanguineous nuclear families used to identify a new locus for recessive non-syndromic hearing loss on 14q. Human Molecular Genetics 4: 1643–8.

Fukushima K, Arabandi R, Srisailapathy CRS, Ni L, Chen A, O'Neill M, Van Camp G, Coucke P, Smith SD, Kenyon JB, Jain P, Wilcox ER, Zbar RIS and Smith RJH. (1995b) An autosomal recessive non-syndromal form of sensorineural hearing loss maps to 3p-DFNB6. Genome Research 5: 305–8.

Garrod AE. (1902) A study in chemical individuality. Lancet II: 1616.

Gibson F, Walsh J, Mburu P, Varela A, Brown KA, Antonio M, Beisel KW, Steel KP and Brown SD (1995) A type VII myosin encoded by the mouse deafness gene shaker-1. Nature 374: 62–4.

Glasscock, ME. (1973) The stapes gusher. Achives of Otolaryngology 98: 82–91.

Goldspiel BR, Green L and Calis KA. (1993) Human gene therapy. Clinical Pharmacy 12: 488–505.

Gold M and Rapin I. (1994) Non-Mendelian mitochondrial inheritance as a cause of progressive genetic sensorineural hearing loss. International Journal of Pediatric Otorhinolaryngology 30: 91–104.

Goodman AC. (1965) Reference zero levels for pure-tone audiometers. ASHA 7: 262–3.

Goodyear R, Holley M and Richardson G (1994) Hair and supporting-cell differentiation during the development of the avian inner ear. Journal of Comparative Neurology 351: 81–93.

Gorlin RJ, Toriello HV and Cohen MM, jr. (1995) Hereditary Hearing Loss and Its Syndromes. New York: Oxford University Press.

Graham JM, Hixon H, Bacino CA, Deack-Hirsch S, Semina E and Murray JC. (1995) Autosomal dominant transmission of a Goldenhar-like syndrome with linkage to the branchio–oto–renal syndrome. Pediatric Research 37: 83A.

Grimberg J, Nawoschik S, Belluscio L, McKee R, Turck A and Eisenberg A. (1989) A simple and efficient non-organic procedure for the isolation of genomic DNA from blood. Nucleic Acids Research 17: 390.

Grisanti G, Crino S and Scilabra JL. (1992) Diagnosi delle sordità genetiche. La Nuova Clinica Otorinolaringolatrica 3: 113–116.

Grisanti G, D'Amico A, Crino S and Scilabra JL. (1996) Artificial intelligence in audiology: an expert system for the diagnosis of genetic syndromes with hearing loss. New Review of Applied Expert Systems 2: 169–183.

Gu Y, Hukriede NA and Fleming RJ (1995) Serrate expression can functionallly replace Delta activity during neuroblast segregation in the Drosophilia embryo. Development 121: 855–65.

Guan MX, Fischel-Ghodsian N and Attardi G. (1996) Biochemical evidence for nuclear gene involvement in phenotype of non-syndromic deafness associated with mitochondrial 12S rRNA mutation. Human Molecular Genetics 5: 963–71.

Guilford P, Arab SB, Blanchard S, Levilliers J, Weissenbach J, Belkahia A and Petit C. (1994a) A non-syndromic form of neurosensory, recessive deafness maps to the pericentromeric region of chromosome 13q. Nature and Genetics 6: 24–8.

Guilford P, Ayadi H, Blanchard S, Chaib H, Le Paslier D, Weissenbach J, Drira M and Petit C. (1994b) A human gene responsible for neurosensory, non-syndromic recessive deafness is a candidate homologue of the mouse sh-1 gene. Human Molecular Genetics 3: 989–93.

Gyapay G, Morissette J, Vignal A, Dib C, Fizames C, Millasseau P, Marc S, Bernardi G,

Lathrop M and Weissenbach J. (1994) The 1993–94 Genethon human genetic linkage map. Nature and Genetics 7: 246–339.

Hall J. (1974) Stickler syndrome presenting as a syndrome of cleft palate, myopia and blindness inherited as dominant trait. Birth Defects Original Article Series 10: 157–71.

Hall JW III and San Agustin TB et al. (1996) Autosomal dominant non-syndromic low-frequency hearing loss in five generations. XXIII International Congress on Audiology, Bari.

Hasson T, Skowron JF, Gilbert DJ. Avraham KB, Perry WL, Bement WM, Anderson BL, Sherr EH, Chen Z-Y, Greene LA, Ward DC, Corey DP, Mooseker MS, Copeland NG and Jenkins NA. (1996) Mapping of unconventional myosins in mouse and humans. Genomics 36: 431–9.

Hayashi JI, Ohta S, Kikuchi A, Takemitsu M, Goto Y and Nonaka I. (1991) Introduction of disease-related mitochondrial DNA deletions into HeLa cells lacking mitochondrial DNA results in mitochondrial dysfunction. Proceedings of the National Academy of Sciences 88: 10614–18.

Heitzler P and Simpson P. (1991) The choice of cell fate in the epidermis of Drosophilia. Cell 64: 1083–92.

Helwig U, Imai K, Schmahl W, Thomas BE, Varnum DS, Nadeau JH and Balling R (1995) Interaction between undulated and Patch leads to an extreme form of spina bifida in doubly mutant mice. Nature and Genetics 11: 60–3.

Holt IJ, Harding AE and Morgan-Hughes JA. (1988) Deletions of muscle mitochondrial DNA in patients with mitochondrial myopathies. Nature 331: 717–19.

Holten A. and Parving A. (1985) Aetiology of hearing disorders in children at the 'schools for the deaf'. International Journal of Pediatric Otorhinolaryngology 10: 229.

Hu DN, Qui WQ, Wu BT, Fang LZ, Zhou F, Gu YP, Zhang QH and Yan JH. (1987) Prevalence and genetic aspects of deaf mutism in Shanghai. Journal of Medical Genetics 24: 589–92.

Huoponen K, Vilkki J, Aula P, Nikoskelainen EK and Savontaus M-L. (1991) A new mtDNA mutation associated with Leber hereditary optic neuroretinopathy. American Journal of Human Genetics 48: 1147–53.

Hutchin T, Haworth I, Higashi K, Fischel-Ghodsian N, Stoneking M, Saha N, Arnos C and Cortopassi G. (1993) A molecular basis for human hypersensitivity to aminoglycoside antibiotics. Nucleic Acids Research 21: 4174–8.

Iannaccone PM and Scarpelli DG. (1993) Exploring pathogenetic mechanisms using transgenic animals. Annals of Medicine 25: 131–8.

ISO 7029. (1984) Acoustics — threshold of hearing by air conduction as a function of age and sex for otologically normal persons. International Organization for Standardization.

Jaber L, Shohat M, Bu X, Fischel-Ghodsian N, Yang HY, Wang SJ and Rotter JI. (1992) Sensorineural deafness inherited as a tissue specific mitochondrial disorder. Journal of Medical Genetics 29: 86–90.

Jacobson J. (1995) Nosology of deafness. Journal of the American Academy of Audiology 6: 80–92.

Jacobson SG, Mohindra J, Held R, Dryja TP and Albert DM. (1984) Visual acuity development in tyrosinase-negative oculocutaneous albinism. Documenta Ophthalmologica 56: 337–44.

Jain PK, Fukushima K, Deshmukh D, Arabandi R, Thomas E, Kumar S, Lalwani AK, Ploplis B, Skarka H, Srisailapathy CRS, Wayne S, Zbar RIS, Verma IC, Smith RJH and Wilcox ER. (1995) A human recessive neurosensory nonsyndromic hearing impairment locus is a potential homologue of the murine deafness (dn) locus. Human Molecular Genetics 4: 2391–5.

Jean-François MJB, Lertrit P, Berkovic SF, Crimmins D, Morris J, Marzuki S and Byrne E. (1994) Heterogeneity in the phenotypic expression of the mutation in the mitochondrial tRNA(LeuUUR)) gene generally associated with the MELAS subset of mitochondrial encephalomyopathies. Australian and New Zealand Journal of Medicine 24: 188–93.

Kadowaki T, Kadowaki H and Mori Y et al. (1994) A subtype of diabetes mellitus associated with a mutation of mitochondrial DNA. New England Journal of Medicine 14: 962–7.

Kafalides NA. (1971) Isolation of collagen from basement membranes containing three identical α chains. Biochemical and Biophysical Research Communications 45: 226–34.

Kajiwara K, Berson EL and Dryja TP. (1994) Digenic retinitis pigmentosa due to mutations at the unlinked peripherin/RDS and ROM1 loci. Science 264: 1604–8.

Kaplan J, Gerber S, Bonneau D, Rozet JM, Delrieu O, Briard ML, Dollfus H, Ghazi I, Durier JL, Frezal J and Munnich A. (1992) A gene for Usher syndrome type 1 (USH1A) maps to chromosome 14q. Genomics 14: 979–87.

Kaplitt MG, Leone P, Samulski RJ, Xiao X, Pfaff DW, O'Malley KL and During MJ. (1994) Long-term gene expression and phenotypic correction using adeno-associated virus vectors in the mammalian brain. Nature and Genetics 8: 148–54.

Karasawa M, Zwacka RM, Reuters A, Fink T, Hsieh CL, Lichter O, Francke U and Weiher H. (1993) The human homolog of the glomerulosclerosis gene MPV17: structure and genomic organization. Human Molecular Genetics 2: 1829–34.

Keithley EM, Ryan AF and Feldman ML. (1992) Cochlear degeneration in aged rats of four strains. Hearing Research 59: 171–8.

Kimberling WJ, Smith SD, Ing PS and Tinley S (1989) A comment on the analysis of families with prelingual deafness. American Journal of Human Genetics 45: 157–8.

Kimberling WJ, Weston MD, Möller C, Davenport SLH, Shugart YY, Priluck IA, Martini A, Milani M and Smith RJH. (1990) Localization of Usher syndrome type II to chromosome 1q. Genomics 7: 245–9.

Kimberling WJ, Möller CG, Davenport S, Priluck IA, Beighton PH, Greenberg J, Reardon W, Weston MD, Kenyon JB, Grunkemeyer JA, Pieke Dahl S, Overbeck LD, Blackwood DJ, Brower AM, Hoover DM, Rowlands P and Smith RJH. (1992) Linkage of Usher syndrome type I gene (USH1B) to the long arm of chromosome 11. Genomics 14: 988–94.

Kingma H. (1997) Clinical testing of the statolith ocular reflex. ORL, in press.

Kingma H, Gulikers H, de Jong I, Jongen R, Dolmans M and Stegeman P. (1995) Real time binocular detection of horizontal, vertical and torsional eye movements by an infra red video–eye tracker. Acta Otolaryngologica 120: 9–15.

Kingma H, Stegeman P and Vogels R. (1997) Static ocular torsion induced by whole body roll and visual stimulation. European Archives of Otorhinolaryngology 254 (Suppl. 1).

Kloepfer HW, Languaite JK and McLaurin JW. (1966) The hereditary syndrome of congenital deafness and retinitis pigmentosa (Usher's syndrome). Laryngoscope 76: 850.

Knowlton RG, Weaver EJ, Struyk AF, Knobloch WH, King RA, Norris K, Shamban A, Uitto J, Jimenez SA and Prockop DJ. (1989) Genetic linkage analysis of hereditary arthro-ophthalmopathy (Stickler syndrome) and the type II procollagen gene. American Journal of Human Genetics 45: 681–88.

Kocher W. (1960) Untersuchungen zur Genetik und Pathologie des Entwicklung von 8 Labyrinth-Mutanten (deaf–walzer–shaker–Mutanten) des Maus (Mus musculus). Z Vererbn 91: 114–40.

Konigsmark BW and Gorlin RJ. (1976) Genetic and Metabolic Deafness. Philadelphia: WB Saunders.

Kotani II, Newton PB III, Zhang S, Chiang YL, Otto E, Weaver L, Blaese RM, Anderson WF and McGarrity GJ. (1992) Improved methods of retroviral vector transduction and production for gene therapy. Human Gene Therapy 5: 19–28.

Kotin RM, Siniscalco M and Samulski RJ et al. (1990) Site-specific integration by adeno-associated virus. Proceedings of the National Academy of Sciences 87: 2211–15.

Kraal B, Zeef LAH, Mesters JR, Boon K, Vorsten-Bosch ELH, Bosch L, Anborgh PH, Parmeggiani A and Hilgenfeld R. (1995) Antibiotic-resistance mechanisms of mutant EF-Tu species in Escherichia coli. Biochemistry and Cell Biology 73: 1167–77.

Kruglyak L, Daly M and Lander E. (1995) Rapid multipoint linkage analysis of recessive traits in nuclear families, including homozygosity mapping. American Journal of Human Genetics 56: 519–27.

Lalwani AK, Walsh BJ, Reilly PG, Muzyczka N and Mhatre AN. (1996) Development of in vivo gene therapy for hearing disorders: introduction of adeno-associated virus into the cochlea of the guinea-pig. Gene Therapy 3: 588–92.

Lander E and Bostein D. (1987) Homozygosity mapping: a way to map human recessive traits with the DNA of inbred children. Science 236: 1567–70.

Lane PW. (1972) Two new mutations in linkage group XVI of the house mouse. Flaky tail and varitint-waddler J. Journal of Heredity 63: 135–40.

Lane PW. (1987) New mutants and linkages: deafwaddler (dfw). Mouse News Letter 77: 129.

Lane PW and Deol MS. (1974) Mocha, a new coat color and behavior mutation on chromosome 10 of the mouse. Journal of Heredity 65: 362–4.

Larget-Piet D, Gerber S, Bonneau D, Rozet JM, Mare S, Ghazi I, Dufier JL, David A, Bitoun P, Weissenbach J, Munnich A and Kaplan J. (1994) Genetic heterogeneity of Usher syndrome type I in French families. Genomics 21: 138–43.

Laroche C and Hétu R. (1997) A study of the reliability of automatic audiometry by the frequency scanning method (Audioscan). Audiology 36: 1–18.

Leib DA and Olivo PD. (1993) Gene delivery to neurons: is herpes simplex virus the right tool for the job? Bioessays 15: 547–54.

Lestienne P and Bataille N. (1994) Mitochondrial DNA alterations and genetic diseases: a review. Biomedicine and Pharmacotherapy 48: 199–214.

Liberfarb RM and Goldblatt A. (1986) Prevalence of mitral-valve prolapse in the Stickler syndrome. American Journal of Medical Genetics 24: 387–92.

Lina-Granade G, Collet L et al. (1996) Age of onset and audiometric configuration in autosomal dominant genetic hearing loss. XXIII International Congress on Audiology, Bari.

Liu XZ, Walsh J, Mburu P, Kendrick-Jones J, Cope MJTV, Steel KP and Brown SDM. (1997) Mutations in the Myosin VIIA gene cause non-syndromic recessive deafness. Nature and Genetics 16: 188–190.

Lowell CA, Soriano P and Varmus HE. (1994) Functional overlap in the src family: inactivation of hck and fgr impairs natural immunity. Genes Development 8: 387–98.

Lyon MF and Searle AC. (eds). (1989) Genetic Variants and Strains of the Laboratory Mouse. Oxford: Oxford University Press.

McCarty DM, Ni TH and Muzyczka N. (1992) Analysis of mutations in adeno-associated virus rep protein *in vivo* and *in vitro*. Journal of Virology 66: 4050–57.

Majumder PP, Ramesh A, and Chinnappan D. (1989) On the genetics of prelingual deafness. American Journal of Human Genetics 44: 86–99.

Martin JAM, Bentzen O, Colley JRT, Hennebert D, Holm C, Iurato S, de Jonge A, McCullen O, Meyer ML, Moore WJ and Morgan A. (1981) Childhood deafness in the European Community. Scandinavian Journal of Audiology 10: 165–74.

Martini A, Cremers C et al. (1996) European Working Group on genetic hearing impairment. XXIII International Congress on Audiology, Bari.

Martinuzzi A. et al. (1992) Correlation between clinical and molecular features in two MELAS families. Journal of Neurological Sciences 13: 222–9.

Meredith R. (1991) Audiometric Identification of Carriers of Non-manifesting Genes for Deafness. MSc Thesis. University of Southampton.

Meredith R, Stephens D, Sirimanna T, Meyer Bisch C and Reardon W. (1992) Audiometric detection of carriers of Usher's syndrome type II. Journal of Audiological Medicine 1: 11–19.

Merrouche Y and Favrot MC (1992) Retroviral gene therapy and its application in oncohematology. Human Gene Therapy 3: 285–91.

Meyer-Bisch C. (1996) Audioscan: a high-definition audiometry technique based on constant-level frequency sweeps — a new method with new hearing indicators. Audiology 35: 63–72.

Meyer zum Gottesberge AM, Reuter A and Weiher H. (1996) Inner ear defect similar to Alport's syndrome in the glomerulosclerosis mouse model MPV17. European Archives of Otorhinolaryngology 253: 470–4.

Michel (1863) Memoire sur les anomalies congenitales de l'oreille interne. Gazette Medicale de Strasbourg 4: 55–8.

Miller SA, Dykes DD and Polesky HF. (1988) A simple salting out procedure for extracting DNA from human nucleated cells. Nucleic Acids Research 16: 1215.

Mitch A and Goldenberg AL. (1996) Mechanisms of muscle wasting. New England Journal of Medicine 335: 1897–1905.

Mochizuki T, Lemmink HH, Mariyama M, Antignac C, Gubler MC, Pirson Y, Verellen-Dumoulin CH, Chan B, Schröder CH, Smeets HJ and Reeders ST. (1994) Identification of mutations in the α3(IV) and α4(IV) collagen genes in autosomal recessive Alport syndrome. Nature and Genetics 8: 77–82.

Mondini C. (1791) Anatomica surdi nati section. De Bononiensi Scientarium et Artium Instituto atque Academia Commentarii. VII: 419–28.

Moraes CT, Ciacci F, Silvestri G et al. (1993) Atypical clinical presentation associated with the MELAS mutation at position 3243 of human mitochondrial DNA. Neuromuscular Disorders 3: 43–50.

Morton NE. (1991) Genetic epidemiology of hearing impairment. Annals of the New York Academy of Sciences 630: 16–31.

Müller M, Smolder JWT, Meyer Zum Gottesberge AM, Reuter A, Zwacka RM, Weiher H and Klinke R (In press) Loss of auditory function in transgenic Mpv17-deficient mice. Hearing Research.

Muzyczka N. (1992) Use of adeno-associated virus as a general transduction vector for mammalian cells. Current Topics in Microbiology and Immunology 158: 97–129.

Myat A, Henrique D, Ish-Horowicz D and Lewis J. (1996) A chick homologue of Serrate and its relationship with Notch and Delta homologues during central neurogenesis. Developments in Biology 174: 233–47.

Nabel E, Pompili V, Plautz G and Nabel G. (1994) Gene transfer and vascular disease. Cardiovascular Research 28: 445–55.

Nance WE, Rose SP, Conneally PM and Miller JZ (1977) Opportunities for genetic counselling through institutional ascertainment of affected probands. In: Lubs HA, de la Cruz F. (eds), Genetic Counselling. New York: Raven Press, pp. 307–32.

Neri G. and Zollino M. (1992) Ipoacusie neurosensoriali dell'infanzia: rischio genetico e sua prevenzione. Otorinolaringoiatria Pediatrica 3: 143.

Newton VE. (1985) Aetiology of bilateral sensorineural hearing loss in young children. Journal of Laryngology and Otology (Suppl.) 10: 1.

Osako S and Hilding DA. (1971) Electron microscopic studies of capillary permeability in normal and Ames waltzer deaf mice. Acta Otolaryngologica 71: 365–76.

Pabla SH, McCormick B and Gibbin K. (1991) Retrospective study of the prevalence of bilateral sensorineural deafness in childhood. International Journal of Pediatric Otorhinolaryngology 22: 161.

Padwa BL, Bruneteau RJ and Mulliken JB. (1993) Association between 'plagiocephaly' and hemifacial microsomia. American Journal of Medical Genetics 47: 1202–7.

Paparella MM. (1985) Sensorineural hearing loss in children-Genetic. In Paparella MM, Shumrick DA eds. Otolaryngology. 3rd ed. Philadelphia, Saunders.

Parkman R and Gelfand E. (1991) Severe combined immunodeficiency disease, adenosinedeaminase deficiency and gene therapy. Current Opinion in Immunology 3: 547–51.

Parving A. (1996) Epidemiology of genetic hearing impairment. In: Martini A, Read A, Stephens D (eds), Genetics and Hearing Impairment. London: Whurr, pp. 73–81.

Parving A, France EA and Stephens SDG. (1996) Factors causing hearing impairment in identical birth cohorts in Denmark and Wales. Journal of Audiological Medicine 5: 67–72.

Phelps PD and Lloyd GAS. (1989) In: Diagnostic Imaging of the Ear (second edition). London: Springer Verlag.

Phelps PD, Reardon W, Pembrey M, Bellman S and Luxon L. (1991) X-linked deafness, stapes fixation and a distinctive defect of the inner ear. Neuroradiology 33: 326–30.

Pieke Dahl S, Kimberling WJ, Gorlin MB, Weston MD, Furman JMR, Pikus A and Möller C. (1993) Genetic heterogeneity of Usher syndrome type II. Journal of Medical Genetics 30: 843–8.

Pietromonaco SF, Denslow DN and O'Brien TW. (1991) Proteins of mammalian mitochondrial ribosomes. Biochimie 73: 827–35.

Poulton J, Morten KJ, Marchington D, Weber K, Brown GK, Rotig A and Bindoff L. (1995) Duplications of mitochondrial DNA in Kearns–Sayre syndrome. Muscle and Nerve 3: S154–58.

Prezant TR, Agapian JV, Bohlman MC, Bu X, Ötzas S, Qiu W-Q, Amos KS, Cortopassi GA, Jaber L, Rotter JI, Shohat M and Fischel-Ghodsian N. (1993) Mitochondrial ribosomal RNA mutation associated with both antibiotic-induced and non-syndromic deafness. Nature and Genetics 4: 289–94.

Probst R, Lonsbury-Martin BL and Martin GK. (1991) A review of otoacoustic emissions. Journal of the Acoustical Society of America 89: 2027–67.

Prochazka M, Leiter EH, Serreze DV and Coleman DL. (1987) Three recessive loci required for insulin-dependent diabetes in non-obese diabetic mice. Science 237: 286–9.

Quick CA, Fish A and Brown C. (1973) The relationship between cochlea and kidney. Laryngoscope 83: 1469–82.

Rao PSS and Inbaraj SG. (1980) Inbreeding effects on fetal growth and development. Journal of Medical Genetics 17: 27–33.

Reardon W. (1992) Genetic deafness. Journal of Medical Genetics 29: 521–6.

Reardon W and Harding AE. (1995) Mitochondrial genetics and deafness. Journal of Audiological Medicine 4: 40–51.

Reid FM, Vernham GA and Jacobs HT. (1994) A novel mitochondrial point mutation in a maternal pedigree with sensorineural deafness. Human Mutation 3: 243–7.

Reid FM, Rovio A, Holt IJ and Jacobs HT. (1997) Molecular phenotype of a human lymphoblastoid cell-line homoplasmic for the np 7445 deafness-associated mitochondrial mutation. Human Molecular Genetics 6: 443–49.

Remes AM, Majamaa K, Herva R and Hassinen IE. (1993) Adult onset diabetes mellitus and neurosensory hearing loss in maternal relatives of MELAS patients in a family with the tRNA mutation. Neurology 43: 1015–20.

Rep M and Grivell LA. (1996) The role of protein degradation in mitochondrial function and biogenesis. Current Genetics 30: 367–80.

Roberts J. (1968) Hearing Status and Ear Examination: Findings among Adults United States, 1960–1962. Report series II, No. 32. Rockville, MD: National Center for Health Studies.

Rolfsen RM and Erway LC. (1984) Trace metals and otolith defects in mocha mice. Journal of Heredity 75: 158–62.

Rolston DW. (1988) Principles of Artificial Intelligence and Expert System Development. New York: McGraw-Hill.

Rosenhall U. (1996) Laboratory evaluation II. Auditory function. In: Baloh R and Halmagyi G. (eds), Disorders of the Vestibular System. New York: Oxford University Press, p. 215.

Roychoudhury AK. (1976) Incidence of inbreeding in different states in India. Demography of India 5: 108–19.

Roychoudhury AK. (1980) Consanguineous marriages in Tamil Nadu. Journal of the Indian Anthropological Society 15: 167–74.

Royden CS, Pirrotta V and Jan LY. (1987) The tko locus, site of a behavioural mutation in *Drosophilia melanogaster*, codes for a protein homologous to prokaryotic ribosomal protein S12. Cell 51: 165–73.

Ruben RJ and Rapin I. (1988) Management of hearing-impaired and deaf infants and children. In: Aberti PW and Ruben RJ (eds). Otologic Medicine and Surgery (Volume II). New York: Churchill Livingstone, pp 1665–94.

Ruben RJ, Van De Water TR and Steel KP. (1991) Genetics of hearing impairment. Annals of the New York Academy of Sciences 630.

Samara G, Sawicki MP, Hurwitz M and Passaro E Jr. (1993) Molecular biology and therapy of disease. American Journal of Surgery 165: 720–7.

Sambrook J, Fritsch EF and Maniatis T. (1989) Molecular Cloning Laboratory Manual (second edition). Cold Spring Harbor, NY: Cold Spring Harbor Laboratory Press.

Samulski RJ, Zhu X, Xiao X, Brook JD, Housman DE, Epstein N and Hunter LA (1991) Targeted integration of adeno-associated virus (AAV) into human chromosome 19. EMBO Journal 10: 3941–50.

Sank D. (1963) Genetic aspects of early total deafness. In: Rainer JD, Altschuler KZ, Kallmann FJ. (eds). Family and Mental Health Problems in a Deaf Population. New York: Colombia University Press, pp. 28–81.

Schenkel J, Zwacka RM, Rutenberg CH, Reuter A, Waldherr R and Weiher H. (1995) Functional rescue of the glomerulosclerosis phenotype in Mpv17 mice by transgenesis with the human MPV17 homologue. Kidney International 48: 80–4.

Schrander-Stumpel CTRM, de Die-Smulders CEM, Hennekam RCM, Fryns JP, Bouckaert PXJM, Brouwer OF, da Costa JJ, Lommen EJP and Maaswinkel-Mooy PD. (1992) Oculoauriculovertebral spectrum and cerebral anomalies. Journal of Medical Genetics 29: 326–31.

Schrott A and Spoendlin H. (1987) Pathology of the Ear. Cambridge, MA: Harvard University Press.

Schuknecht HF (1973) Pathology of the Ear. Cambridge, MA: Harvard University Press.

Shoffner JM, Lott MT, Lezza AM, Seibel P, Ballinger SW and Wallace DC. (1990) Myoclonic epilepsy and ragged-red fiber disease (MERRF) is associated with a mitochondrial DNA tRNALys mutation. Cell 61: 931–7.

Shoffner JM and Wallace DC. (1995) Molecular analysis of oxidative phosphorylation diseases for detection of mitochondrial DNA mutations. In: Dracopoli NC, Haines JL, Korf BR, Moir DT, Morton CC, Seidman CE, Seidman JG and Smith DR (eds), Current Protocols in Human Genetics. New York: John Wiley, pp. 9.9.1–24.

Shortliffe EH (1976) Computer based medical consultations: MYCIN, New York, Elsevier.

Sirimanna T, France L and Stephens D. (1994) Alport's syndrome: can the carriers be identified by audiometry? Clinical Otolaryngology 20: 158–63.

Sirimanna T, Stephens D and Board T. (1996) Tinnitus and audioscan notches. Journal of Audiological Medicine 5: 38–48.

Smith C. (1953) The detection of linkage in human genetics. Journal of the Royal Statistical Society B15: 153–84.

Smith RJH. (1986) Medical diagnosis and treatment of hearing loss in children. In: Cummings CW, Fredrickson JM, Harker LA, Krause CJ and Schuller DE. (eds), Otolaryngology–Head and Neck Surgery. St. Louis, MS: CV Mosby.

Smith RJH, Lee EC, Kimberling WJ, Daiger SP, Pelias MZ, Keats BJB, Jay M, Bird A, Reardon W, Guest M, Ayyagari R and Hejtmancik JF. (1992) Localization of two genes for Usher syndrome type I to chromosome 11. Genomics 14: 995–1002.

Smith RJH, Berlin CI, Hejtmancik JF, Keats BJB, Kimberling WJ, Lewis RA, Möller CG, Pelias MZ and Tranebjærg L. (1994) Clinical diagnosis of the Usher syndromes. American Journal of Medical Genetics 50: 32–8.

Smith-Thomas LC, Kent C, Mayer RJ and Scotting PJ. (1994) Protein ubiquitination and neuronal differentiation in chick embryos. Developments in Brain Research 81: 171–7.

Steel KP and Brown SDM. (1994) Genes and deafness. Trends in Genetics 10: 428–35.

Steel KP, Barkway C and Bock GR. (1987) Strial dysfunction in mice with cochleo-saccular abnormalities. Hearing Research 27: 11–26.

Stefanelli M. (1988) Strutturazione del ragionamento medico. Medicina ed Informatica 5: 78–85.

Stephens D and Francis M. (1996) The detection of carriers of genetic hearing loss. In: Martini A, Read A and Stephens D. (eds), Genetics and Hearing Impairment. London: Whurr, pp. 100–108.

Stephens D, Meredith R, Sirimanna T, France L, Almqvist C and Haugen H. (1995) Application of the audioscan in the detection of carriers of genetic hearing loss. Audiology 34: 91–7.

Stevenson AC and Cheeseman EA. (1956) Hereditary deaf mutism, with particular reference to Northern Ireland. Annals of Human Genetics 20: 177–231.

Stickler GB and Pugh DG. (1967) Hereditary progressive arthro-ophthalmopathy. II. Additional observations on vertebral abnormalities, a hearing defect, and a report of a similar case. Mayo Clinic Proceedings 42: 495–500.

Stickler GB, Belau PG, Farrell FJ, Jones JD, Pugh DG, Steinberg AG and Ward LE.

(1965) Hereditary progressive arthro-ophthalmopathy. Mayo Clinic Proceedings 40: 433–55.

Stolbova D and Valvoda M. (1985) Detection of normal hearing carriers of the gene for autosomal dominant progressive sensorineural hearing loss. Acta Otolaryngologica 99: 509–15.

Strachan T and Read AP. (1996) Human Molecular Genetics. New York: Wiley.

Street VA, Robinson LC, Erford SK and Tempel BL. (1995) Molecular genetic analysis of distal mouse chromosome 6 defines gene order and positions of the deafwaddler and opisthotonos mutations. Genomics 29: 123–30.

Sutphen R, Galan-Gomez E, Cartada X, Newkirk PN and Kousseff BG. (1995) Tracheo-oesophageal anomalies in oculoauriculovertebral (Goldenhar) spectrum. Clinical Genetics 48: 66–71.

Tamagawa Y, Kitamura K, Ishida T, Ishikawa K, Tanaka H, Tsuji S and Nishizawa M. (1996) A gene for a dominant form of non-syndromic sensorineural deafness (DFNA11) maps within the region containing the DFNB2 recessive deafness gene. Human Molecular Genetics 5: 849–52.

Timms AR, Steingrimsdottir H, Lehmann AR and Bridges BA. (1992) Mutant sequences in the rpsL gene of *Escherichia coli* B/R — mechanistic implications for spontaneous and ultraviolet-light mutagenesis. Molecular and General Genetics 232: 89–96.

Tiranti V, Chariot P, Carella F, Toscano A, Soliveri P, Girlanda P, Carrara F, Fratta GM, Reid FM, Mariotti C and Zeviani M. (1995) Maternally inherited hearing loss, ataxia and myoclonus associated with a novel point mutation in mitochondrial tRNA$^{ser(UCN)}$ gene. Human Molecular Genetics 4: 1421–7.

Tokahashi M and Hokunan K. (1992) Localization of type VI collagen and laminin in the guinea pig inner ear. Annals of Otology Rhinology and Laryngology 191: 58–62.

Tranebjaerg L. (1996) Genetic Causes of Syndromic and Non-syndromic Hearing Loss. Status and Clinical Consequences. Budapest: III Eufos.

Tryggvason K, Zhou J, Hostikka SL and Shows TB. (1993) Molecular genetics of Alport syndrome. Kidney International 43: 38–44.

Tzagoloff A and Myers AM. (1986) Genetics of mitochondrial biogenesis. Annual Review of Biochemistry 55: 249–85.

Usher CH. (1914) On the inheritance of retinitis pigmentosa, with notes of a case. Royal London Ophthalmogical Hospital Reports 19: 130–236.

Van Camp G, Smith RJH. Hereditary hearing loss homepage. ⟨http://alt.www.uia.ac.be/u/dnalab/hhh.html⟩

Van Camp G, Coucke P, Kunst D, Schatteman I, Van Velzen D, Marres H, van Ewijk M, Declau F, Van Hauwe P, Meyers J, Kenyon J, Smith S, Smith R, Djelantik B, Cremers C, Van de Heyning P and Willems P. (1997) Linkage analysis of progressive hearing loss in five extended families maps the DFNA2 gene to a 1.25 Mb region on chromosome 1p. Genomics, in press.

Van den Ouweland JMW, Lemkes HHP, Ruitenbeek W, Sandkuijl LA, Devijlder MF, Stuyvenberg PA, Van de Kamp JJP and Maasen JA (1992) Mutation in mitochondrial transfer RNA(Leu(UUR)) gene in a large pedigree with maternally transmitted type-II diabetes mellitus and deafness. Nature and Genetics 1: 368–71.

Van den Wijngaart WSIM and Verschuure J et al. (1985) Follow up study in a family with dominant progressive hereditary sensorineural hearing impairment. I. Analysis of hearing deterioration. Audiology 24: 233–40.

Van Rijn R. (1994) Torsional Eye Movements in Humans. Thesis. University of Maastricht.

Wagenaar M, Snik AFM, Kimberling WJ and Cremers CWRJ. (1996) Carriers of the Usher syndrome type I: is audiometrical identification possible? American Journal of Otolaryngology 17: 853–8.

Wallace DC. (1992) Diseases of the mitochondrial DNA. Annual Review of Biochemistry 61: 1175–1212.

Wallace DC, Singh G, Lott MT, Hodge JA, Schurr TG, Lezza AMS, Elsas LJ and Nikoskelainen EK. (1988) Mitochondrial DNA mutation associated with Leber's hereditary optic neuropathy. Science 242: 1427–30.

Wayne S, Lowry RB, McLeod DR, Kraus R, Farr C and Smith RJH. (1997) Localization of the Usher Syndrome type 1F (Ush 1F) to chromosme 10. American Journal of Human Genetics 61(Suppl): A300.

Wayne S, Der Kaloustian VD, Schloss M, Polomeno R, Scott DA, Hejtmancik JF, Sheffield VC and Smith RJH. (1997) Localization of the Usher syndrome type ID gene (USH1D) to chromosome 10. Human Molecular Genetics (in press).

Webster DB. (1985) The spiral ganglion and cochlear nuclei of deafness mice. Hearing Research 18: 19–27.

Weeks DE, Ott J and Lathrop GM (1990) SLINK: a general simulation program for linkage analysis. American Journal of Human Genetics 47: A204.

Weidauer H and Arnold W. (1976) Strukturelle Veränderungen am Hörorgan beim Alport syndrome. Zeitschrift Laryngologica Rhinologica Otologica 55: 6–16.

Weiher H. (1993) The glomerulosclerosis in transgenic mice: the gene and its human homologue. In: Grånfeld JP, Bach JF, Kreis H, Maxwell MH (eds), Advances in Nephrology. St Louis, MS: CV Mosby, pp. 37–42.

Weiher H, Noda T, Gray DA, Sharpe AH and Jaenisch R. (1990) Transgenic mouse model of kidney disease: insertional inactivation of ubiquitously expressed gene leads to nephrotic syndrome. Cell 62: 425–34.

Weissenbach J, Gyapay G, Dib C, Vignal A, Morissette J, Millasseau P, Vaysseix G and Lathrop M. (1992) A second-generation linkage map of the human genome. Nature 259: 794–801.

Weil D, Blanchard S, Kaplan J, Guilford P, Gibson F, Walsh J, Mburu P, Varela A, Levilliers J, Weston MD, Kelley PM, Kimberling WJ, Wagenaar M, Levi-Acobas F, Larget-Plet D, Munnich A, Steel KP, Brown SDM and Petit C. (1995) Defective myosin VIIA gene responsible for Usher syndrome type 1B. Nature 374: 60–61.

Weil D, Kussel P, Blanchard S, Levy G, Levi-Acobas F, Drira M, Ayadi H and Petit C. (1997) The autosomal recessive isolated deafness, DFNB2 and the Usher IB Syndrome are allelic defects of the myosin VIIA gene. Nature Genetics 16: 191–193.

Williams DA. (1990) Expression of introduced genetic sequences in hematopoietic cells following retroviral-mediated gene transfer. Human Gene Therapy 1: 229–39.

Winter RB and Baraitser M. (1993) Multiple Congenital Anomalies. A Diagnostic Compendium. London: Chapman & Hall.

Zee DS and Hain TC. (1993) Otolith-ocular reflexes. In: Sharpe JA, Barber HO (eds), The Vestibulo-ocular Reflex and Vertigo. New York: Raven Press, pp. 69–78.

Zlotogora J, Sagi M, Schuper A, Leiba H and Merin S. (1992) Variability of Stickler syndrome. American Journal of Medical Genetics 42: 337–9.

Zwacka R, Reuter A, Pfaff E, Moll J, Gorgas K, Karasawa M and Weiher H. (1994) The glomerulosclerosis gene MPV17 encodes a peroxisomal protein producing reactive oxygen species. EMBO Journal 13: 5129–34.

Index